FAMILY DISEASES
ARE YOU AT
RISK?

FAMILY DISEASES

ARE YOU AT

RISK?

BY MYRA VANDERPOOL GORMLEY

Genealogical Publishing Co., Inc.

This book summarizes recent findings in the field of medical genetics and explains how standard genealogical practices may be used in compiling a family health history; however, it is not intended to replace the services of a family physician. The author and publisher disclaim responsibility for any adverse effects resulting from the information presented in this book and urge you to consult a physician before drawing any conclusions about your family health history.

Genograms of the Adams family and Thomas Jefferson's family, which appear in chapter 4, are reprinted from *Genograms in Family Assessment,* by Monica McGoldrick, M.S.W., and Randy Gerson, Ph.D., by permission of W.W. Norton & Company, Inc. Copyright © 1985 by Monica McGoldrick and Randy Gerson.

Dedicated to my mother,

Doris Fricks Vanderpool

Contents

Foreword

Researchers from the Harvard Medical School in Boston and Molecular Therapeutics, Inc., in West Haven, Connecticut, reported independently this spring that they have identified the mechanism by which cold viruses enter cells. They believe they know what to do to develop a drug that will prevent the common cold.

Myra Vanderpool Gormley is probably not stunned by this news, even though chief executives and employers throughout the world may well be dancing in their accounting departments. Genetic engineering, genetic screening, and genetics-based drug therapy, Gormley writes, promise the elimination or control of more than 3,000 diseases and disorders caused by defective genes or chromosomes.

Gormley is a family historian. For decades she has urged us to discover, through genealogy, our individualities and our strong commonalities. But the idea of genetics has been in her mind all along. She recalls a physician's question about her mother's glaucoma. She recalls the concerns of repeated generations: should cousins marry? The Amish and the Mormons ask her about intermarriage. She recalls the Daughters of the American Revolution opening their files of 200,000 irrefutable pedigrees to study.

Gormley's faithful pruning of countless family trees gives a special resonance to this extraordinary book, which is a carefully researched guide to the diseases that plagued our ancestors, the transmission of those diseases from generation to generation, and the treatments, cures, and long-term hopes offered by medical genetics.

Gormley knows that a job applicant's history of cancer, as an example, has enabled some employers to reject their application out of hand. She even knows of a firm that offers employers genetic screening programs to root out "bad gene" applicants. In this groundbreaking work, however, she traces the scientific revolution that could eliminate this kind of discrimination once and for all. Her contents page alone is a message of hope.

Jean Sharley Taylor
Associate Editor
LOS ANGELES TIMES
March 1989

Preface

We are living in the midst of a medical revolution that has
enormous implications for mankind generally and for you
personally. While geneticists have long been interested in
genealogy and genealogists in genetics, only recently have the two fields
become linked in a way that promises dramatic advances in our understanding of the relationship between genetic disorders and ancestry. This
book is an effort to explore that relationship, to alert you to things you
and your family ought to know about both your family tree and genetic
research, and to examine the scientific breakthroughs that have made
possible much more effective control and treatment of inherited disease.

There are few families who are not affected in some way by genetic
disorders, whether a crippling and devastating disease like cystic fibrosis,
a chronic condition like high blood pressure, or a predisposition to
alcoholism or mental illness. Heart disease, diabetes, and cancer all tend
to "run in families." Yet few of us know much about genetic disorders
— what they are, how they are transmitted, how they may be screened
or treated, or even how to find information on them. Indeed, few of us
know whether we or our children are at risk from such disorders.

As a writer and genealogist, and one concerned about the health of
family members, I was very enthusiastic when my editor at the *Los
Angeles Times* suggested several years ago that I write an article on
genetically transmitted diseases. When I discovered there was no
layman's guide on the subject and that there were in fact virtually no
easily understood materials geared to the non-scientific community, I set
out to expand the article and write a book to fill the void.

Here, in plain language but unstinting detail, is the result of that labor. The product of extensive research as well as deep commitment, *Family Diseases: Are You at Risk?* will, I hope, answer your questions, offer you insights and perhaps assurances, and, most of all, provide you with knowledge and information that will be beneficial to you and your family. We stand on the brink of so many wonderful and practical applications of a genealogically enhanced genetics that it has never been more important to be familiar with your family's medical history and the means at hand to protect your family's health.

I am indebted to many who aided my research and who shared their family stories about genetic disorders. I especially want to thank Julia M. Case for her diligent assistance and constant encouragement, and the following who helped me in various ways I regret I cannot adequately acknowledge in this short space: Susan E. King, Marianne Shaw Montgomery, Jo White Linn, Persis Reynolds Shook, Jean Nooner Strode, Mary Powell Gorham, Janet Nixon Baccus, Johni Cerny, Howard L. Nurse, Jone Carlson, Mary McCampbell Bell, Dort F. Tikker, Ralph Crandall, Dr. Jay Sacks, Laura McCoy Herbert, Sylvia Seelig Woods, Gary Boyd Roberts, Carmen Ulmer, Director of Communications for Southern California March of Dimes Chapter, Birth Defects Foundation, and Brett Emerson of the National Center for Education in Maternal and Child Health in Washington, D.C. My work would have been much diminished without the cooperation of staff members of the numerous genetic foundations and organizations who so graciously supplied me with information.

Finally, a special thanks to my husband, Leo C. Gormley, without whose support and encouragement I would never have been able to undertake, let alone complete, this project.

Myra Vanderpool Gormley

FAMILY DISEASES
ARE YOU AT
RISK?

1 — The Genetics Revolution and You

If you are like most people, you probably think that genetic diseases are rare. While it is true that *each* of the more than 3,000 genetic disorders is relatively rare, taken as a group they are quite common. Innumerable people suffer from disorders due wholly or in part to defective genes or chromosomes. Genetic diseases are far more prevalent than is generally realized, as the statistics below indicate:

- 12 to 15 million Americans have a genetic disorder of one kind or another.

- 20 million Americans are carriers of true genetic defects.

- One out of every 250 newborn babies has a genetic disorder.

- One out of every three babies or young children admitted to a hospital is there because of a genetic problem.

- Each of us carries an average of between four and seven abnormal recessive genes.

Moreover, it is now recognized that the major cripplers and killers of adults — diabetes, heart disease, various psychiatric illnesses, and some cancers — all have significant genetic components. Obviously, then, we all have a tremendous stake in the outcome of current research in the field of human genetics. Fortunately, that research is blazing frontiers almost undreamed of just a generation ago. Hardly a day goes by that one does not read in a newspaper or magazine about some new discovery or breakthrough. In fact, it can be said that nothing less than a revolution is occurring in our understanding of human genetics. The new developments promise to reduce the prevalence of genetic disorders and improve and prolong the lives of their victims. Among the recent advances: more and better tests for prenatal diagnosis; improved technology to sustain the lives of seriously ill and deformed newborns and increase the life expectancy of people afflicted by genetic disorders; and the capacity to undertake mass screenings to identify carriers of harmful genes.

This genetics revolution is already affecting your life, whether you realize it or not. The family doctor who once took your family health history by asking what childhood diseases you had and whether your parents or grandparents had suffered from diabetes or heart disease, has expanded the medical pedigree with questions about your ethnic origins, dates and causes of death of all four grandparents, and the kinds of diseases suffered by other relatives.

An increasing number of knowledgeable people are seeking information about their genetic makeup and risks. As a result of heightened public awareness, there has been a growing demand for genetic services. Thirty years ago, for example, there were a mere handful of genetic counseling centers, but by 1983 there were more than 500 in the national listing of Clinical Genetic Service Centers. Even persons who were adopted and who are facing reproductive decisions are demanding changes in adoption procedures to insure the adoptee's access to his or her genetic history.

The new human genetics is revolutionizing medical research. It is providing precise information on who is most vulnerable to what kind of illness and who particularly should avoid certain environmental agents. It is helping researchers design more effective and less harmful drugs, and it is providing fresh insights into the function of regulatory genes that affect all human growth and development, from birth to death.

Such major illnesses as heart disease, cancer and schizophrenia, each of which probably involves many different genes, are too complex to yield their secrets even to the new sophisticated tests and therapies. However, some multi-gene diseases may be prevented or lessened in severity by means of drugs, or by manipulating lifestyle or other environmental variables. As scientists discover the genetic risk factors of certain diseases, people who find out that they are susceptible may be able to reduce their chances of illness simply by altering specific aspects of their behavior and environment. As research advances, it is enabling doctors to help millions of people prevent or control inherited diseases, including some diseases that have been identified only in the last twenty years.

With these new prospects and opportunities also come new problems and dilemmas. For example, the increased life expectancy for children with such genetic conditions as Down's syndrome, sickle-cell anemia, hemophilia and cystic fibrosis has overtaxed the existing social services of many communities, and yet the affected individuals and their families desperately need these services. Similarly, current research on familial patterns in behavior disorders is providing insight into the possible inheritance of certain psychiatric disorders, not only schizophrenia but a whole range of dysfunctions — a promising development, to be sure, but one also fraught with troublesome consequences. Early identification, by reviewing family history, of relatives who are at risk of developing similar behavioral disorders may allow interventions to prevent the more severe manifestations of the diseases, but it may also prematurely or needlessly bring a latent condition to the surface and in any case would likely entail costly long-term therapy.

Your family physician has marvelous new tools and data at his disposal for the early diagnosis and treatment of genetic disease, but his success in handling a particular case depends in large measure on the patient's own assistance in acquainting him with the family's health background. Few people, however, are able to give their doctors a comprehensive family health briefing, simply because they have limited knowledge themselves of the family's medical pedigree. If your grandparents died before you were born or while you were small, you may have no idea what diseases caused their deaths, and recollections by other family members may be faulty or not entirely forthright. Most of us are not sufficiently knowledgeable about the medical histories of our other relatives — even of our brothers and sisters. And just knowing the cause of death of family members is not enough, for your grandfather may have died of what was termed "old age" on his death certificate, but he may also have suffered from diabetes or arthritis, which may have been the primary reason for his decline.

Determining a genetic link for a disease can be extremely complex, especially where one inherits the disorder through a recessive gene. Individuals affected with a recessive disease will often find no pattern or precedent for the disease in their family history. While you yourself may not suffer any medical problems stemming from it, if your spouse also carries the same recessive gene, then the disorder can manifest itself in your children or show up in your grandchildren if your children's spouses also have the same recessive gene.

Many developmental anomalies, birth defects, and disease processes simply seem to "run in families" without being associated with predictable high-recurrence risks. These disorders are referred to as "multifactorial" traits since several factors, both genetic and environmental, are involved in their etiology.

Chromosomal abnormalities comprise another classification of genetic disorders. Some of these may be inherited with a high-recurrence risk, and only through chromosomal analysis of the affected individual and appropriate relatives can persons be identified who may be unaffected carriers capable of passing on the abnormality.

In X-linked (sex-linked) diseases, the characteristic pedigree pattern is that of one or more affected males in multiple generations who are related through apparently normal female carriers — persons who can transmit a genetic disease to their children, but who are not ill with the disease themselves. Hemophilia is an example of this type of X-linked disease. Carrier females are at a 25-percent risk of having affected male children, and all daughters of affected males are obligate carriers. However, some family structures are such that the gene may have been passed through several unaffected females and, by chance, not inherited by their sons.

In the diagnosis of any genetic disorder it helps to have as detailed a family history as possible. For example, if you are of Jewish origin, your doctor should know whether you descend from Sephardic, Oriental or Ashkenazi ancestors, as there are genetic diseases that are characteristically found in one group and not in the others. Frequently it is necessary to examine numerous members of the patient's family before diagnosis of a genetic disorder can be made with certainty. And today, with families scattered throughout the country — even the world — it is unlikely your family doctor would be able to do this; which makes a thorough, documented family health history all the more valuable to you and your relatives. In addition to enhancing the accuracy of diagnosis, a complete family health history also is necessary for effective genetic counseling. Such counseling concerns itself not only with the question of the probability of other family members being affected, but also with aspects of prognosis, treatment, and emotional adjustment. Effective counseling can be achieved only with a full medical history of the family.

A good family health history should include information about you, your siblings, your children and your ancestors and their siblings. If you are female, your doctor will probably ask you questions about any abortions, stillbirths, miscarriages, children who died during infancy and members of the sibship who have died. A thorough prenatal history is crucial if you are starting your own family. This should include mention of any use of drugs, consumption of alcohol, and exposure to various infectious diseases. You should always be concerned about the presence of congenital anomalies in your family as well as the clustering of any traits or diseases, and tell your doctor about them.

Knowledge of the ethnic background of your family, as well as the place of birth of parents, grandparents, and occasionally great-grandparents, is obviously relevant and important information. The places of their births should include not only the country but also the city or region, and when available the name of the hospital. However, few except experienced genealogists can answer all these questions.

Let me offer an example here to illustrate how beneficial the task of reconstructing a family's history can be. An avid genealogist friend called me one day to see if I knew anything about the migration patterns of Italians or the Spanish to Ireland and Scotland, where most of her family had originated. Her six-week-old grandson had been diagnosed as having thalassemia major, and the doctors wanted complete information about the child's family tree.

Thalassemia is a hereditary form of anemia, occurring most often in people of Mediterranean descent. Causing enlargement of the spleen, iron accumulation in the tissues, respiratory difficulties, and retarded growth and development, it is a serious disease with no known cure. The only treatment for it requires repeated transfusions, and hence is complicated, painful and costly. "I need to know if any of my Scotch-Irish families might have had roots in the Mediterranean, especially Italy," my friend said. She had been unable to find any connection but thought perhaps there had been some migration from the Mediterranean area to the British Isles. So began a search into a pedigree that had been traced to Ireland and Scotland on the maternal side, with very little known about the paternal line of the child. His genealogist grandmother searched diligently to pinpoint the origins of the family, but despite her efforts she could turn up no known connection to any places in the Mediterranean. All of her and her husband's families had come from the British Isles as far back as they could determine. Information about the paternal ancestry of the child also revealed only northern European roots.

The child's doctor continued to believe he suffered from thalassemia, and recommended that all the maternal family members be tested for the disorder. However, on the basis of the good genealogical data provided by the maternal grandmother on the origins of both families involved, they decided to re-test the child, and thereby discovered that an error in the interpretation of the original test had been made. By being able to rule out thalassemia, the doctors then were able to identify and treat the child's illness.

Family history encompasses more than genealogy, which is simply the tracing of descent. It includes genealogical charts and lineages, but more broadly, it is the story of one's ancestors —in effect, the sum of their biographies. Today genealogists themselves are more interested in family histories than in bare birth, marriage and death records. They recognize the importance to their clients of including information about the health of ancestors, realizing that while material gathered today may not be of immediate significance, its long-term value could be incalcul-able. As the science of genetics becomes even more refined in future years, comprehensive and well-documented family health histories will be a boon to your grandchildren and great-grandchildren and later generations in their quest for good health.

In 1984 the largest hereditary society in the nation, the 200,000-plus-member National Society of the Daughters of the American Revolution (DAR), launched a Family Tree Genetics project in conjunction with Vanderbilt University's School of Medicine at Nashville, Tennessee. The DAR donated $50,000 for the computer software for the study and its members submitted thousands of five-generation medical-genealogi-cal charts. Sarah Hughey King, then president-general of the DAR and the leading force behind the project, urged members to participate because "early diagnosis of glaucoma, diabetes, growth hormone deficiency, Huntington's disease, cancer, circulatory disorder, dyslexia and Alzheimer's, to name only a few [genetic diseases], makes it possible to treat and, in many instances, prevent problems for future generations." "We are fortunate," she observed, "in that we know whence we came. Our research will serve as an inspiration to others." Under the directorship of Dr. John A. Phillips III of the Division of Genetics at Vanderbilt, the research and tabulation of the DAR members' medical genealogies has continued, with the results scheduled to be published in the near future.

It is believed that genetic factors may be involved in 25 percent of diseases. Frightening as this figure is, many genetic disorders once thought to be incurable can now be controlled or treated successfully if they are diagnosed *early*. Family health histories can provide descendants with an invaluable tool, alerting them to watch for early warning signs of such illnesses as breast cancer, diabetes, and glaucoma. By compiling a family health tree, you can provide clues to medical problems that have plagued your families for generations, and you can alert your descendants to potential health problems — even before symptoms appear. If there are genetic disorders in your family, they can be diagnosed and treated in light of current scientific knowledge. Given the pace of the genetics revolution, you may find that you are able to minimize or prevent some illnesses that doomed family members in the past.

The recent wave of genetic research has already brought about the following discoveries:

- There is a widespread genetic defect which may explain why up to 10 percent of whites in North America and Europe do not properly metabolize certain drugs. It is estimated that between 35 and 43 percent of the white population of North America and Europe carry at least one copy of this mutant gene. A recent study involving the drug debrisoquine, which is used to control high blood pressure, revealed this metabolic abnormality. It is a recessive gene, but this genetic trait affects the metabolism of more than twenty commonly prescribed drugs, including antidepressants, antiarhythmics (which smooth out irregular heartbeat) and the cough suppressant dextromethorphan.

- Researchers have recently developed a blood test to identify children at risk of retinoblastoma (fatal eye tumors). This disease is highly curable if treated before it has spread outside the eye. Identification of the relevant gene means a blood or tissue test can be given to those who have developed the disease as children and want to know their risk of passing the gene on.

• Scientists have developed a simple blood test to diagnose alcoholism that may also offer a way to screen people to see if they have inherited a risk of becoming alcoholic.

• Researchers have determined that bad habits and bad genes that lead to obesity and heart disease in adulthood can be identified and controlled as early as infancy. This is significant since high blood pressure and high cholesterol levels in infants have been found to persist throughout childhood, if not corrected, and long-term dietary patterns appear to fall into place by age two.

• While still a long way from solution, sickle-cell anemia and Cooley's anemia — both blood diseases common in Greeks, Italians and others of Mediterranean descent —may some day be treatable as a result of work now in progress. California scientists have developed a faster method to detect the defective genes responsible for the disorders.

• Scientists have reported promising preliminary results of a new method of predicting Down's syndrome risk by analyzing a family's genes. This discovery could ultimately prevent as many as 30 percent of such births.

• Researchers have discovered the genetic defect that causes phenylketonuria, a rather uncommon genetic disease that can lead to mental retardation. If the disease is diagnosed early enough the retardation can be entirely prevented by careful control of diet.

• A study of manic-depressive disease in three generations of a family has shown for the first time that defective genes can cause psychiatric disorders. Previous studies have suggested that genetics could contribute to such disorders, but this new finding is the first demonstration of a genetic defect in a mental disease that shows no anatomical abnormalities in the brain. This study traced the defective gene through three generations of an Old Order Amish family in southeastern Pennsylvania. Members of the family who inherited the gene had an 85-percent chance of suffering manic-depression or related conditions during their lifetime.

- Doctors are able to use a new genetic test to tell couples what their chances are of having a child with Duchenne muscular dystrophy, an always-fatal disease. The new technique can also track through families the faulty genes that cause cystic fibrosis and ten other inherited diseases. Baylor College of Medicine in Houston and the Children's Hospital in Boston are now routinely offering this test.

- The National Institute of Mental Health reports that scientists have identified the genetic defect responsible for Gaucher's disease, a rare disorder that most commonly affects Jews of Eastern European descent. The encouraging findings should improve testing for the disease and may eventually lead to a treatment.

- A study of genes from eighty-two members of a family in Iceland, of whom twenty-one had a rare form of cleft palate or a related birth defect, showed the faulty gene lies on a portion of the X chromosome. This discovery in turn may lead to a better understanding of another birth defect, spina bifida, which is in some cases also linked to the X chromosome.

- Research continues on human gene therapy in which doctors transplant copies of a normal gene into the cells of a patient whose own body lacks the gene or has it in an abnormal form. Eventually this process may be used to cure patients with cystic fibrosis, various forms of hemophilia, and possibly muscular dystrophy.

- Utah researchers have devised a genetic test for a kidney disease that affects some 400,000 Americans and is responsible for one in ten kidney dialysis patients. Though still in a preliminary stage, the test would enable doctors to diagnose the disease before symptoms appear, which is usually in middle age. The affliction, known as polycystic kidney disease, is a dominant disorder, meaning that those who carry the disease gene will pass it on to half of their children, who will then develop the condition.

- Swedish researchers have found that men whose mothers died of stroke face three times the usual risk of dying of the same disease and that men are at increased risk of stroke if they are overweight. The same study found high blood pressure is clearly linked with stroke and also has a possible genetic connection.

Impressive as they are, these developments represent only the leading edge of a genetics revolution that is likely to have exponentially more far-reaching results. Within the next ten years, between 2,000 and 3,000 genetic markers will be identified that could lead to predictive tests for thousands of illnesses, from stroke to heart attack to cancer to Alzheimer's disease.

You can't pick your genes — or change them, yet — but knowing which family health problems are likely to have been passed on to you and your descendants can alert you early enough to prevent many of them or minimize their effects. Knowing that a certain disease runs in your family may mean you will have to make adjustments in your eating habits or take appropriate medications or have more frequent checkups. Or you may find your risk of a certain disease is not as high as you feared. In addition, many other conditions, though not inherited in the way genetic diseases are, do tend to occur more frequently in some families than in others, and by researching your family health tree you will be alerted to these also. Those with serious genetic illnesses in their background will find full information about them helpful in deciding (perhaps with the aid of genetic counseling) whether or not to have children. Family medical information gathered now and incorporated in your family history can help young and still unborn generations take advantage of future medical discoveries.

You may uncover some frightening things in your family's medical past. However, you are just as likely to discover that you come from hardy, long-lived stock. Regardless of what you find, you can use that information to improve the health care of your loved ones. And what better legacy to leave your descendants than a family health tree with its valuable clues to good health?

In order to compile a medical pedigree, you need to know what genetic disorders are and how they are transmitted, so you will recognize and understand them as they apply to your family. This will be discussed in the next chapter.

2 — What are Genetic Diseases?

A genetic disease is an illness or condition traceable to one's genetic makeup. You probably know that hemophilia, sickle-cell anemia and cystic fibrosis are such diseases, but did you know that obesity, some forms of cancer, some forms of early heart disease, and some blindness, deafness and birth defects are inheritable? All told, more than 3,000 genetic conditions have been identified. Some are very rare, but others, such as diabetes, are among the most common illnesses.

Genes are the chemical information we inherit from our parents at the moment we are conceived. They determine our biological "constitution." Genes cause us to be similar to our parents, and they control how we grow and what we look like. They also make us resistant to some illnesses and prone to others.

Each of us carries some faulty genes. Some genetic diseases are caused by a single faulty gene in one affected parent. However, most disorders occur only if both parents transmit the same faulty gene. Fortunately, this happens only rarely.

Genetic diseases are passed from generation to generation the same way brown eyes and dimples are. Some genetic problems are present at birth — they are congenital — but many, such as adult-prone diabetes, do not show up until later in life. There is no immunity against genetic illness, and when a disease is caused by a faulty gene, there is always some risk that it will recur in a family, though the chance may be less than is feared.

Genetic diseases also may be caused by a chromosome defect affecting a specific pregnancy. The cells composing all organisms contain a fixed number of chromosomes, occurring in pairs. In normal humans there are 23 pairs or a total of 46 chromosomes per cell. Important exceptions are the reproductive cells (sperm and ovum), each containing 23 unpaired chromosomes. At conception, each parent provides one reproductive cell; as the sperm and egg fuse, they form a single cell with a full chromosome count.

Genetic conditions are inherited. Therefore, knowing which diseases exist in a particular family is important to your doctor to aid him or her in arriving at the right diagnosis and in preventing or treating symptoms. Living with a hereditary condition becomes the concern of the entire family.

Types of Inheritance of Genetic Disorders

There are four mechanisms by which genetic defects may be transmitted from one generation to another: (1) autosomal dominant inheritance, where the trait is inherited from one parent and from the previous generation; (2) recessive inheritance, where both parents are unaffected; (3) X-linked (or sex-linked) inheritance, in which the gene for the characteristic is known to be on the X chromosome; and (4) multifactorial inheritance patterns.

Autosomal Dominant Inheritance — Autosomal means that the gene pair is present in a chromosome pair other than the sex chromosomes. In dominant inheritance an affected child usually has a parent with the same disorder. When the parent has a dominant gene for a disease, there is a 50-percent risk that *each* child will manifest the defect, though it may not be evident at birth. There is an equal likelihood that a child will *not* receive the abnormal gene, and thus that child and his or her children should be free of the defect.

There are about 2,000 confirmed or suspected autosomal dominant disorders. Examples are:

- Huntington's disease (Huntington's chorea)

- polydactyly (extra fingers or toes)

- achondroplasia (a form of dwarfism)

- chronic simple glaucoma (some forms)

- hypercholesterolemia (high blood cholesterol levels, with propensity to heart disease)

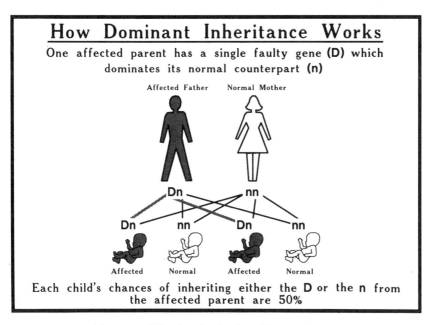

How Dominant Inheritance Works

One affected parent has a single faulty gene **(D)** which dominates its normal counterpart **(n)**

Affected Father   Normal Mother

Dn   nn

Dn   nn   Dn   nn

Affected   Normal   Affected   Normal

Each child's chances of inheriting either the **D** or the **n** from the affected parent are 50%

(Courtesy of Kingdom Productions, Houston, Texas.)

Recessive Inheritance — Both parents of an affected child appear essentially normal, but by chance both may carry the same harmful gene, although neither may be aware of it. The child who receives the defective gene from both parents may have a significant birth defect. Recessive inherited diseases tend to be severe and often cause death early in life. When both parents are carriers of a harmful recessive trait, each of their children will run a 25-percent (one-in-four) risk of manifesting that genetic disease, and each has a fifty-fifty chance of receiving only a single defective gene and becoming a clinically normal carrier of the genetic trait like the parents. The chance of inheriting a recessive disorder is increased in a child whose parents are "blood" relations (consanguineous).

There are more than 1,000 confirmed or suspected autosomal recessive disorders, which include:

- cystic fibrosis

- galactosemia

- phenylketonuria

- sickle-cell disease

- thalassemia

- Tay-Sachs disease

- Gaucher's disease

Note: Parents who have one child affected by a disorder due to a recessive inheritance may think that a 25-percent, or one-in-four, risk means that the next three children are not endangered. THIS IS NOT TRUE. The risk of genetic disease is the same for every child of the same mother and father.

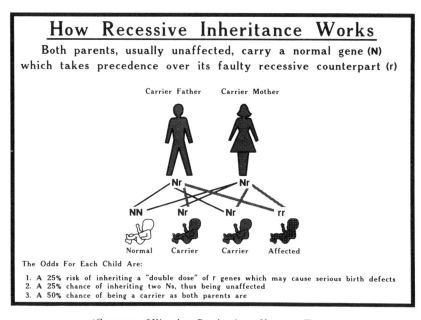

How Recessive Inheritance Works

Both parents, usually unaffected, carry a normal gene (N) which takes precedence over its faulty recessive counterpart (r)

Carrier Father   Carrier Mother

Nr   Nr

NN   Nr   Nr   rr

Normal   Carrier   Carrier   Affected

The Odds For Each Child Are:

1. A 25% risk of inheriting a "double dose" of r genes which may cause serious birth defects
2. A 25% chance of inheriting two Ns, thus being unaffected
3. A 50% chance of being a carrier as both parents are

(Courtesy of Kingdom Productions, Houston, Texas.)

X-Linked Inheritance (also called sex-linked) — Normal females have two X chromosomes. Normal males have one X and one Y. In X-linked inheritance, a clinically normal mother carries a faulty gene on one of her X chromosomes. In such cases, each son has a fifty-fifty risk of inheriting that gene and manifesting the disorder. Each of her daughters has an equal chance of being a carrier like her mother, and is usually unaffected by the disease, but is capable of transmitting it to *her* sons. No male-to-male transmission of X-linked disorders can occur — that is, a father cannot pass the disorder on to his son.

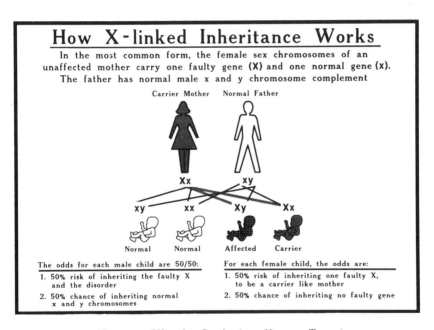

How X-linked Inheritance Works

In the most common form, the female sex chromosomes of an unaffected mother carry one faulty gene (**X**) and one normal gene (**x**). The father has normal male x and y chromosome complement

Carrier Mother   Normal Father

Xx   **xy**

xy   xx   **Xy**   **Xx**

Normal   Normal   Affected   Carrier

The odds for each male child are 50/50:
1. 50% risk of inheriting the faulty X and the disorder
2. 50% chance of inheriting normal x and y chromosomes

For each female child, the odds are:
1. 50% risk of inheriting one faulty X, to be a carrier like mother
2. 50% chance of inheriting no faulty gene

(Courtesy of Kingdom Productions, Houston, Texas.)

There are some 250 confirmed or suspected disorders transmitted by a gene or genes on the X chromosome. Examples are:

- color blindness
- hemophilia
- agammaglobulinemia (lack of immunity to infections)
- muscular dystrophy (some forms)
- spinal ataxia (some forms)

Multifactorial Inheritance — The pattern of transmission in this group is less well-defined, but these genetic disorders result from the interaction of many genes with other genes or with environmental factors. With one affected child in a family, chances of other children having the same defect are 5 percent or less. The number of defects due to multifactorial inheritance is unknown. However, some that are thought to be multifactorial include:

- cleft lip and/or palate

- clubfoot

- congenital dislocation of the hip

- spina bifida

- hydrocephalus (water on the brain, occurring with spina bifida)

- pyloric stenosis (narrowed or obstructed opening from the stomach into the small intestine)

- congenital heart defects

- diabetes mellitus (abnormal sugar metabolism)

Who is Affected

Certain genetic diseases are widespread in the population; others affect primarily certain ethnic or racial groups. Cystic fibrosis is one of the most common genetic diseases among Americans because it mainly affects whites of northern and western European ancestry. Tay-Sachs is a recessive-gene disorder that often strikes infants of Central and Eastern European Jewish descent. Cooley's anemia (a form of thalassemia) affects mainly people of Mediterranean descent, while sickle-cell anemia is found mainly in blacks.

Some Disorders "Run in Families"

The major diseases that strike American families today — heart disease, cancer and diabetes — all show some tendency to "run in families." This does not mean you are doomed to have one of them if a parent or uncle suffered from the condition, but you should be aware of the risks where there is a precedent for the disease in your family.

Numerous studies have revealed that early heart attacks do run in families. If a person under fifty-five has a relative who had a heart attack before reaching sixty-five, his or her risk of also having one before sixty-five is five to seven times the normal risk for their sex. Moreover, some of the leading factors known to contribute to coronary disease — high cholesterol levels, high blood pressure, diabetes and obesity — have been found to have a genetic link.

Several types of cancer are known to be directly inherited, such as retinoblastoma of the eye. But there also common forms of cancer that tend to run in families, such as cancer of the stomach, endometrium (uterine lining), lung, colon and bladder, breast cancer and malignant melanoma of the skin.

Researchers have established recently that you are likely to develop Type II, or non-insulin-dependent diabetes, the most common form of this disease, if one or both parents have this type. Genetics plays a lesser role in Type I, or insulin-dependent diabetes.

Some Common Genetic Disorders

Obesity and High Blood Pressure — Recently a key study by Dr. Albert J. Stunkard of the University of Pennsylvania demonstrated that obesity is primarily a product of our genes, not our diets. Stunkard concluded that members of obese families have to be even more careful about diet than the rest of the population. Most of us have made this assumption on our own, but we now have scientific evidence to support it.

In another study, Dr. Michael Horan of the National Heart, Lung and Blood Institute found that about half of all fifty-year-olds with high blood pressure have close relatives with high blood pressure. It is also known that diet and obesity play a part in hypertension, but, again, genetics is a key influence. An inborn inability to metabolize sodium is one suspected culprit in genetic hypertension. About half of hypertensives are sensitive to sodium.

Since hypertension can trigger heart attack or stroke and lead to kidney disorders, Horan says persons with hypertensive relatives should "be compulsive" about having their blood pressure checked regularly and work to keep their weight down. There is no evidence that obesity causes hypertension, but weight loss will lower pressure. Keeping blood pressure at a sensible level by weight reduction, diet and, for some, low sodium intake, may even eliminate the need for medication.

Cancer in Families — Cancer of the breast and colon and certain forms of skin cancer are most heavily influenced by family history. Most women are aware that breast cancer runs in families. An American woman normally runs a 6-percent risk of developing breast cancer by age seventy-three. However, if her mother and sister, or two sisters, were victims, the odds increase. But the risks vary according to when and how the disease struck. If the cancers occurred before menopause and in both breasts, the risks are much higher than if they occurred after menopause, in a single breast.

About one-fourth of colon cancer cases appear to be hereditary. Many of these result from a condition called familial polyposis, which is an inherited tendency to form benign intestinal growths that may later become malignant. Members of families with a predisposition to colon cancer should have annual internal examinations for polyps, as well as perform self-administered slide examinations for blood in the stool. Benign polyps should be removed promptly.

About 10 percent of the time, malignant melanoma (the fast-spreading and virulent skin cancer) has been found to cluster in families. Most high-risk families share a tendency to develop moles and growths. If you have a family history of melanoma, you should examine yourself frequently for evidence of change in moles, and have a head-to-toe examination for new growths conducted by a dermatologist.

Inherited cancers, fortunately, seem to be site-specific, meaning that a history of breast cancer, for example, increases the risk of that form of disease but *not* other forms of cancer.

Diabetes — The diabetes that affects middle-age persons — known as non-insulin dependent diabetes or adult-onset diabetes — has a strong family link. Studies have shown there is a one-in-two risk of being affected if you have a parent or sibling who is diabetic, and an even higher risk if both of your parents were diabetic.

About 75 to 80 percent of older diabetics are obese, and some geneticists believe this is because adult-onset diabetics inherit a defect in their fat cells. Persons with a known family history of this disorder are advised to control their weight, exercise regularly, follow a balanced diet and have regular physical examinations, including urine and blood tests.

Osteoarthritis and Osteoporosis — Osteoarthritis, the kind of arthritis caused by wear-and-tear on the body, has not been shown to be family-related, except in one form: Heberden's nodes, which affects the finger joints and is passed from mother to daughter. If you are female and your mother had gnarled or twisted fingers after age fifty, the chances are that you will develop them, too. However, this condition need not be painful or limit joint function.

Osteoporosis, which occurs in women after menopause and causes bone shrinkage, is believed to have a genetic component. If this disorder occurs in your family your doctor will probably recommend that you follow a preventive course, beginning when you are young, by eating a diet rich in calcium.

Eye Disorders — most of the serious eye problems that cause impaired vision in older persons do tend to have strong family connection. These include glaucoma, cataracts and macular degeneration, a condition that damages the eye's fine-vision capability and causes almost 8,000 Americans a year to be classified legally blind.

Glaucoma is readily treatable, but it is a major cause of vision loss in people over age fifty. It can be detected with a simple test and controlled in the overwhelming majority of cases with daily use of eyedrops. Cataract removal is now a commonly performed operation, but early detection is important.

The genetics of eye problems are still unclear, and risks to individual family members have not yet been calculated with any precision. However, if you are middle-age or older and have a single relative afflicted with any of these conditions, you may be at risk and should have a yearly eye examination, including a check for fluid pressure.

Hearing Loss — Some families seem to have more than their share of hearing loss. If your father or mother could not hear well, you may be at risk and should make it a point to have your hearing tested regularly.

One form of hearing impairment that does have a proven hereditary basis is otosclerosis. This disorder occurs when small bones within the ear become fused and prevent normal eardrum movement. The condition develops gradually, and victims may not be aware of a problem until it is advanced. However, otosclerosis can be corrected surgically. Persons with relatives who have the condition should undergo regular hearing tests themselves.

Other Genetic Disorders

Malignant Hyperthermia (MH) — This most often affects Caucasians of northern European heritage, usually older children and young adults. Although both sexes are equally at risk for MH, it occurs more often in males than in females.

In one well-documented case, researchers traced the disease through descendants of French-born Michel Dupuis, who came to Nova Scotia with his wife, Marie Gauterot, in 1651. The Dupuis family tree, meticulously compiled, includes some 4,000 members stretching back to 1642. The founding couple and their offspring farmed in northern Quebec and in southwestern Ontario and intermarried with the Comartin and Caza families. In the mid-1950s descendants of these families began to die unexpectedly during surgery, suggesting a common syndrome related to the administration of anesthesia.

MH was found to be a hereditary condition in which very high body temperatures and muscle rigidity occur when the affected person is exposed to certain anesthetics. It is a genetic defect that alters the way muscles use calcium. For the most part, this defect is benign — some carriers never suffer from it — but in some cases the administration of the most commonly used anesthetics triggers catastrophic chemical changes that make the patient's temperature soar, often to 110 degrees or higher, causing massive damage to the heart, liver, brain and other major organs. Thus, anesthesia, one of medicine's great life-saving tools, for some members of this Dupuis family is a killer.

In addition to French Canadians, families of central European, Italian, Norwegian and Welsh descent suffer from the disease. It is rarely found among blacks or Japanese. In the general population it is roughly estimated that one in 15,000 people carry the hidden disease.

Retinoblastoma — A rare and often hereditary eye cancer that develops in children. This causes diminished vision and retinal detachment, and abnormal pupillary reflexes are common. Left untreated, it can be fatal.

Joseph Disease — In this fatal genetic disorder, loss of specific brain cells leads to paralysis.

Duchenne Muscular Dystrophy — This is an X-linked recessive disease (affecting only males) with symptoms first appearing around the age of three or four. There is progressive wasting of leg and pelvic muscles, followed by confinement to a wheelchair (usually by age twelve), then death, usually from heart disorders, often by age twenty. A group of scientists led by Louis Kunkel of Boston Children's Hospital has identified the gene that, when defective, causes Duchenne MD. The discovery may lead to an effective treatment, even a cure, for the crippling and usually fatal disorder that afflicts 200,000 people in the United States, most of them young boys.

Gaucher's Disease — This is a rare, familial disorder in which defective fat metabolism leads to spleen and liver enlargement and abnormal bone growth. Mortality is high in early childhood, but those who survive through adolescence may live for many years. The genetic mutation for type I is carried by one in 600 Jews of Eastern European ancestry. Work is under way on development of a gene therapy to treat Gaucher's disease.

Huntington's Disease (Chorea) — This abnormal hereditary condition is characterized by progressive chorea (involuntary, rapid, jerky motions) and mental deterioration, leading to dementia. Symptoms usually first appear in the third or fourth decade of life and progress to death, often within fifteen years. As many as 100,00 Americans now living were born to Huntington parents before the parents themselves knew they had the disease. There is no cure, but a genetic test developed at The Johns Hopkins Hospital can identify parents who are carriers and those who are not.

Hurler's Syndrome — In this hereditary disease (autosomal recessive), mucopolysaccharides (any group of complex carbohydrates that are structural parts of connective tissue) and lipids (greasy organic compounds which are stored in the body and serve as energy reserves) accumulate in the tissues and cause mental retardation, enlarged liver and spleen, enlarged head and low forehead. It usually leads to death in childhood from cardiac or pulmonary complications.

Porphyria — This name is given to any of several inherited disorders characterized by dysfunction of the metabolism or porphyrins (any of a number of pigments widely distributed in living tissue), affecting primarily the liver or bone marrow. The affected person excretes large amounts of porphyrins in the urine and suffers from photosensitivity, neuritis and mental disturbances. King George III of Britain had this genetic disorder and for many years was labelled variously as a manic-depressive and "mad." This is a dominantly inherited disease and, because the royal family's genealogy has been well documented, the condition has been traced back to Mary Queen of Scots and down to people living today, over a period of thirteen generations and 400 years in the royal houses of Stuart, Hanover and Prussia. It has been referred to as the "Royal Malady."

Hemophilia — Another disease associated with royalty, this is an inherited disorder characterized by excessive bleeding and occurs almost exclusively in males. England's Queen Victoria, the daughter of Edward, Duke of Kent, was a carrier of this X-linked recessive gene, and it has shown up in many of her descendants.

Marfan's Syndrome — An inherited abnormality (autosomal dominant disorder) characterized by elongation of bones, especially the arms, legs, fingers and toes; joint hypermobility; and abnormalities of the eyes (e.g., dislocation of the lens) and circulatory system. It is suspected that Abraham Lincoln, our twelfth president, had this disorder, and recently there was a diagnosis of this disease in a seven-year-old boy whose lineage was traced back to the great-great-grandparents of the president.

Hereditary Ataxia — This is the name given to a group of degenerative brain and spinal chord conditions shown to be inherited. It is thought that the gene or genes responsible for ataxia cause the body to produce an abnormal protein, which for some unknown reason causes the nerve cells to degenerate, thereby reducing nerve signals to the muscles. Dominant ataxia is passed on as a dominant hereditary disease, with symptoms usually appearing between ages twenty and forty. In the case of Friedreich's ataxia, a recessive form of the disease, the recessive gene may lie dormant for generations until suddenly two people with the defective gene have children. In these instances the symptoms usually appear in childhood or during the teenage years.

An estimated 150,000 people in the United States are affected by the hereditary ataxias. The National Ataxia Foundation, in Wayzata, Minnesota, sponsors research into all forms of ataxia as well as closely related conditions, such as peroneal muscular atrophy (Charcot-Marie-Tooth disease), hereditary spastic paraplegia, ataxia telangiectasia and hereditary tremor, a common neurological disorder.

Abetalipoproteinemia — This rare, inherited metabolic disorder is characterized by severe deficiency or total absence of betalipoproteins (one of the components of cholesterol), abnormally low cholesterol levels, and the presence of abnormal red blood cells. Symptoms include malnutrition, growth retardation, degeneration of the retina and progressive neurological dysfunction.

Asthma — A respiratory disorder characterized by recurrent episodes of breathing difficulties. It is most common in childhood, occurring more often in boys, and has a strong hereditary factor.

Phenylketonuria — A liver enzyme deficiency, this is a rather uncommon genetic disorder that can cause mental retardation. If the disease is diagnosed early enough retardation can be prevented by careful control of the diet.

Galactosemia — This inability to metabolize milk sugar is an autosomal recessive disorder.

Seeking Genetic Counseling

If any of these genetic disorders, or others, occur in your family you may wish to seek genetic counseling. The March of Dimes Birth Defects Foundation recommends you seek genetic counseling if:

- You or your family members have a disease with a genetic component.
- You are a member of an ethnic group with a high risk of certain genetic diseases.
- You have produced an affected child.
- You are an expectant mother thirty-five years of age or older.

For information on genetic counseling see chapter 9.

3 — Is Your Family at Risk?

Few of us know much of anything about our relatives' medical histories, even though such knowledge can play a crucial role in our own health care. More than 3,000 of the 10,000 known diseases and conditions have a strong hereditary component. These include Huntington's chorea and sickle-cell anemia, diabetes, hypertension and heart disease. New ones are being added to the list every day: Alzheimer's, multiple sclerosis, peptic ulcers, schizophrenia, depression, and cancers of the colon, breast, and retina. Researchers have recently found that children whose fathers are alcoholics are four times as likely as other people to become alcoholics and children of people with duodenal ulcers are three times as likely also to suffer ulcers.

What good does it do to know if you are at risk? People who know about a predisposition toward a disease can do a lot to prevent that disease, either by changing high-risk behavior or by detecting health problems early. If you are alerted to the genetic liabilities you carry, you can develop corrective habits, or at least be treated at the earliest possible stage.

A growing number of family practitioners recognize that a detailed family medical history can be valuable both in treating an individual's ailments and in discovering how family psychological patterns influence each member's physical and mental health. Families often pass intact collections of genes from one generation to the next; a marker may be associated with a disease, not necessarily because it is actually involved in causing the disease, but because it sits close to a dangerous gene and is passed on with it. Because of this familial linkage, physicians who are aware of the importance of prediction are beginning to pay closer attention to the family histories they take. No longer does a complete physical examination merely attempt to pinpoint someone's condition at a particular place and time; now it is equally important to find out about heredity, to discover the way genes might run through generations. Markers within families can ease the anxiety of those who might not be at risk and focus attention on those who are.

Some Diseases for Which Genetic Tests are Now Available

—Adult polycystic kidney disease

—AAT deficiency(emphysema)

—Fragile X syndrome

—Sickle-cell anemia

—Duchenne muscular dystrophy

—Cystic fibrosis

—Huntington's disease

—Hemophilia

—Phenylketonuria

—Retinoblastoma

On the Horizon

—Hypertension

—Dyslexia

—Hardening of the arteries

—Cancer

—Manic depression

—Schizophrenia

—Juvenile diabetes

—Familial Alzheimer's

—Multiple sclerosis

—Myotonic muscular dystrophy

The incidence of family-linked diseases is so very great that few of us can afford to remain uninformed on the subject. The rest of this chapter, therefore, focuses on the risks posed by a broad range of genetic disorders.

Heart Disease

Numerous studies have shown a tendency for early heart attacks to "run in families." Doctors say that if a person under fifty-five has a relative who had a heart attack before reaching sixty-five, his or her risk of repeating the relative's experience is five to seven times the normal risk for the person's sex. Some children are born with inherited heart malformations, missing coronary vessels or vessels easily clogged by cholesterol. There is also a genetic component in some of the physical problems that can lead to heart attack, such as high cholesterol levels, high blood pressure, diabetes and obesity.

If no parent, grandparent, aunt or uncle has suffered a heart attack before age 65 and among your close blood relatives no serious high blood pressure, diabetes or high cholesterol exists, and if you are a non-smoker, or quit more than five years ago, your risk of heart disease is low — assuming your lifestyle habits are excellent also.

Your age, sex and genetic makeup influence your susceptibility to heart disease, and these factors are out of your control. However, many major factors that lead to coronary problems are within your control. Both health and behavioral habits may determine whether or not you will suffer a heart attack. For example, if you are overweight, have high blood cholesterol, smoke, do not exercise, drink too much, and overreact to regular tensions and stresses in your life, you are a prime candidate for heart disease. But these undesirable traits can be altered.

Stroke

Every year an estimated 400,000 people in the United States suffer a stroke and about 160,000 of them die soon afterward. Stroke is our third leading killer, after heart disease and cancer, but it is often preventable. A family history of stroke places you at greater risk because it suggests you might have a genetic propensity towards a weakness of the blood vessels.

Being overweight, eating too much sodium, getting too little calcium, overreacting to stress, drinking too much alcohol and having a family history of stroke are all risk factors for development of primary hypertension. Except for family history, these risk factors are due to lifestyle and can be changed. Even if there are family precedents, however, it is possible that your ancestors also had unhealthy lifestyle habits, in which case it is the transmission of those habits rather than genes that put you at risk.

Cancer

Several types of cancer, such as retinoblastoma and colon cancer in families with polyposis (colon polyps that often become malignant), are known to be inherited. There are also other forms of cancer that run in families: cancer of the stomach, endometrium (uterine lining), lung, colon and bladder, breast cancer and malignant melanoma of the skin.

The tendency of cancers to run in families actually goes beyond those specific cancers for which genetic markers have been found. In general, relatives of people who contract cancer are more likely to get the disease themselves. In the normal population, 30 percent of cancer patients have one close relative who also has cancer; 20 percent have two such relatives; and 7 percent have three or more. Leukemia, the cancer of the bone marrow that seems to attack mostly young children, gives an identical twin odds of one in five of contracting the disease if his or her twin has it. Among other siblings, the odds are smaller, but the connection is clear. You perhaps have read about parents who find all their children developing leukemia — a phenomenon that, in the general population, would occur in about one family in a billion if it were by chance.

People who are under sixty years of age and have low levels of pepsinogen 1 carry a risk of stomach cancer that is twenty times higher than that of the general population. Successful treatment of stomach cancer depends partly on catching it early enough. The discovery of the pepsinogen 1 marker should at least give those at risk a better chance of being diagnosed early.

One family whose records were published by the National Cancer Institute illustrates the extent to which familial tendencies can occur. The first patient to be identified as a cancer victim was a woman who had cancer of the cervix. Subsequently, her brother had cancer of the colon, her sister had cancer of the breast, and two nephews contracted a rare and fatal cancer of the blood. Later, three of her six children developed leukemia, as did several distant relatives.

The evidence is overwhelming, then, that if you have a parent, aunt, uncle, grandparent or sibling who had cancer, or one or more other close relatives with cancer, it places you in a higher risk category.

Be sure to alert your doctor to any history of the following cancers, as they appear to run in families.

- Breast cancer
- Colon cancer
- Lung cancer
- Prostate cancer
- Cervical cancer
- Uterine and ovarian cancer
- Skin cancer/melanoma
- Pancreatic cancer
- Kidney cancer

Breast cancer — This has long been observed to run in families. On the average, a woman whose family has experienced at least two cases of breast cancer has a lifetime susceptibility of one in six. If those family members are closely related (your mother and sister, for instance), the odds go up to a very frightening one in three. Since there seems to be a genetic susceptibility toward breast cancer, a mother or sister with breast cancer is your most serious risk factor for developing the disease.

Skin cancer — People with red hair and fair skin, especially when exposed to excessive sunlight, have been found to be prime candidates for skin cancer. The Irish and others of Celtic origin are particularly susceptible. Several other genetic diseases linked with skin cancer also involve increased sensitivity to radiation. One, called xeroderma pigmentosm (XP), causes freckling, reddening, blistering and a tendency to scar when the skin is exposed to sunlight. People with XP must be extra careful about exposure to strong or prolonged sunlight. If you have a pigmented mole, always burn easily and severely, or have a light complexion with blue or light-colored eyes, you should use your common sense about sun-bathing and consult your doctor as a precaution before spending any extended time in the sun.

Kidney cancer — A marker has been found for tumors of the kidneys. It is significant only in cancer-prone families. One patient's family health history turned up ten victims out of forty members of a three-generation family.

Connected Chromosomal Abnormalities — Most cancers are joined by a common thread — they develop in response to some kind of abnormality in chromosomes or genes. Some of the more striking chromosomal abnormalities have long been tied to cancer:

- Children born with Down's syndrome are more prone to leukemia than others.

- Females with Klinefelter's syndrome (an extra X chromosome added to the normal XX complement of sex chromosomes) tend to have an increased chance of contracting breast cancer.

- Those missing a piece of chromosome 13 almost invariably develop cancer of the eye.

- People with the so-called Philadelphia chromosome have higher odds of contracting leukemia.

Diabetes

Researchers have established that one's likelihood of developing Type II, or non-insulin-dependent diabetes, the most common form of the disease, is substantially increased if one or both parents have this type. Also, if one or more grandparents had adult-onset diabetes, or a brother or sister has it, you are at a higher risk.

However, even if there are such precedents in your family, you will not necessarily contract the illness. Many doctors believe the genetic aspect may be kept dormant if you follow a healthy diet, control your weight and exercise regularly.

Although heredity plays an important part in determining who gets diabetes, there is no clear pattern of inheritance, and no exact predictions can be made as to how the disease will appear in future generations. Parents of a diabetic child often wonder how their child can possibly have developed diabetes if there is no history of it on either side of the family. However, we don't always know the medical histories of all of our ancestors. It may be that somewhere in the family tree diabetes did appear, but it may have gone undiagnosed.

Where the hereditary factor comes into play in non-insulin-dependent diabetes, obesity is believed to be the single most important cause. As one doctor put it bluntly, "If you want to avoid diabetes, don't get fat." When there is a family history of obesity and diabetes, if one family member is overweight and another is not, the obese member is more likely to develop the disease.

Huntington's Disease

This is a hereditary disorder of the central nervous system which affects movement, mood and mentation. Hallmarks of the disorder are uncontrollable movements (chorea), intellectual impairment and, in some patients, profound emotional disturbance, especially depression. It is inherited in an autosomal dominant mode with the age of onset usually between 35 and 45, though in 10 percent of the cases it can occur before age 20 and in some instances after the age of 60. Mood or personality changes and minor involuntary movements may precede diagnosis by ten years or more.

A major breakthrough has been made in HD research recently. A DNA marker for the HD gene was found in 1983 by Dr. James Gusella of the Massachusetts General Hospital in Boston. This marker will make it possible to offer a pre-symptomatic test to at least a portion of those at risk of HD. With this new discovery, within families with enough living members to make linkage studies possible, researchers may be able to tell with a high degree of certainty (approximately 95 percent) which individuals have inherited HD and which have not. Initially, the test will be given only to at-risk adults, but prenatal testing has been available since the fall of 1986 at the Johns Hopkins Hospital in Baltimore and the Massachusetts General Hospital to those who live within a 150-mile radius.

For most families, the test will require blood samples from at least two relatives and the person being tested. Obviously, the subject's parents are most important here, but grandparents from the family with a history of HD are also excellent candidates. The subject's brothers, sisters, uncles and aunts (especially unaffected at-risk individuals who are age fifty or older) may also be needed. If either parent is deceased, other family members on both sides become even more crucial to the success of the testing process.

In case there are family members who have HD and are very sick or are old and near death, a program exists to store blood samples. Then if someone passes away, the genetic information from their blood can still be obtained whenever necessary.

Between 60 and 80 percent of the 100,000 Americans at risk of Huntington's say they would like to take advantage of the new test to plan for the future. Others believe, however, that uncertainty is better than the despair that would come from knowing that they carry the defective gene. A recent article in the science magazine *Discover* notes that many of those who previously had said they would take advantage of such a test have not done so. Only a small percentage of the 1,500 persons at risk for the disease in New England had gone in for preliminary counseling by June 1987.

Osteoporosis

If you are female, of northern European ancestry, with fair skin, red or blond hair and small bones, and you have a blood relative who had osteoporosis, lost height, developed dowager's hump or broke a hip, you are at a high risk for osteoporosis. Heredity plays an important primary role in the development of osteoporosis because it influences bone density and hormonal actions, keys to the disease. You are at highest genetic risk of osteoporosis if you are a woman whose mother suffered from it. Additionally, if your physical characteristics fit the profile and if any of your close relatives — aunts, uncles or grandparents — had the disease, consider yourself at high risk.

Cystic Fibrosis

Cystic fibrosis (CF) is the number one genetic killer of children. It takes more lives than juvenile diabetes and muscular dystrophy combined. CF is a debilitating disease inherited from parents with recessive genes and results in the body producing abnormal amounts of thick, sticky mucus that clogs the lungs and pancreas, interfering with breathing and digestion. CF is characterized by the following symptoms: persistent cough, recurrent wheezing, having pneumonia more than once, excessive appetite but poor weight gain, salty-tasting skin and bulky, foul-smelling stools. CF is diagnosed by measuring salt content in sweat.

Approximately 30,000 people in the United States have cystic fibrosis, and it occurs in approximately one in every 2,000 births.

The occurrence of CF is worldwide, yet there are some racial groups in which it is rarely seen or has never been reported. CF occurs much less frequently among black and Asian populations, for example.

An estimated twelve million Americans (one in twenty) are unknowing, symptomless carriers of the gene that causes CF. There is no cure, although medication and exercise can relieve serious symptoms, sometimes enabling victims to survive to age thirty-five or so. However, the average lifespan is twenty-one years.

Presently the CF Foundation is on the brink of developing a screening program for the entire U.S. population that would allow it to specifically identify the twelve million carriers. This screening effort would be the largest in medical history. Whether or not an unborn child has the disease can be detected with about 95 percent accuracy by testing fetal cells for markers, but the analysis currently is only attempted for couples who already have a child with cystic fibrosis.

People frequently are surprised to discover that the CF gene runs in their family and that they have a greater-than-average risk of bearing a child with CF. In fact, in the great majority of cases where a child is diagnosed with CF, it is often the first time in the family's recollection that a family member has ever had cystic fibrosis. However, when CF occurs, both sides of the family are involved. Since the parents received their genes from their parents, at least one of the grandparents on each side of the family of a CF victim must carry the defective gene. Therefore, although CF may not have occurred in any other family members, the gene for CF had to be present in the family tree.

Sickle-Cell Anemia

Sickle-cell anemia is a hereditary blood disease that affects more than two million persons worldwide. The disease is believed to have originated in Africa thousands of years ago and most of the two million afflicted today are African. In addition, an estimated 25 percent of the continent's 200-million population are genetic carriers of the disease. In the United States some 50,000 to 100,000 blacks have the disease and more than two million are carriers (about 7 to 9 percent of the nation's total black population). The disease is also found in the West Indies, Central and South America, the Middle East, the Mediterranean region and as far east as India. Interestingly, these are all areas where malaria has at one time been quite prevalent. Most cases in the U.S. occur among blacks and Hispanics of Caribbean ancestry. The disease also affects some people of Arabian, Greek, Maltese, Sicilian, Sardinian, Turkish, and southern Asian ancestry.

Carriers of a single gene for the disease are called sickle-cell trait individuals. They, for the most part, have normal health and are unaware that they carry a genetic defect. However, people who inherit two genes are most often severely afflicted with the life-shortening condition.

Hemophilia

Hemophilia is a hereditary blood-clotting disorder which affects males almost exclusively. Although it is inherited, the disorder occurs occasionally in families without a known history of the disease. It can occur in any family, and affects people of all races and nationalities.

The clotting disorders included in the term hemophilia are Hemophilia A (classical hemophilia, Factor VIII deficiency) and Hemophilia B (Christmas disease, Factor IX deficiency). Von Willebrand's disease (which also affects females) and other rare clotting disorders may have similar symptoms, but they are not usually termed hemophilia. Still, all of these disorders are included within the programs of the National Hemophilia Foundation. There are about 20,000 males in the United States with hemophilia, which occurs in one out of every 4,000 live male births. The figures for von Willebrand's disease appear to be comparable.

Ulcers

Twenty million Americans have duodenal ulcers. Duodenal ulcers were one of the first disorders to have a genetic marker, mainly because testing for the marker — ABO blood type — has always been so simple. The major ABO types have been known since 1900, and comprehensive statistics on all sorts of ethnic, racial and geographical groups have been compiled through their identification. Forty-four percent of white Americans have blood type O, compared to only 25 percent of Pakistanis and more than 85 percent of Chippewa Indians. Blood type O points to a slight, but significant, predisposition to duodenal ulcers; those who have it are 1.4 times as likely to get ulcers as those with types A, B or AB.

Studies have shown that it can be predicted that individuals in certain families have two chances in five of contracting duodenal ulcers. Members of families with a history of the disorder are usually advised to reduce their chances of getting ulcers by avoiding certain foods, coffee and alcohol, and by staying away from the light midnight snacks that stimulate the stomach to produce digestive juices without giving it enough material to digest.

Pernicious Anemia

Pernicious anemia is a rare but identifiable genetic disorder. It occurs when the red blood cells lack a specific protein that allows them to absorb vitamin B12. The cells need the vitamin; without it, they become bloated and heavy. Ultimately their inefficiency can disrupt the function of peripheral nerves, resulting in severe neurologic problems. The disorder strikes only about one out of every 200 older women of Scandinavian, Irish and English descent. Its tendency to run in families and the presence of a defective protein makes it likely that investigators will soon discover a causative genetic marker that can pinpoint those at risk.

Hunter's Syndrome

A genetic disease caused by deficiency of the enzyme iduronate sulfatase, its most common features are joint stiffness, dwarfing, and coarse facial features. Progressive mental deterioration also occurs, but the severity varies. This is an X-linked recessive trait. Mildly affected patients may lead relatively normal lives and survive into their sixties, while those with a severe case may die in their early teens.

Hurler's Syndrome

This is an autosomal recessive disease caused by deficiency of the enzyme alpha-L-iduronidase. It is a severe, progressive disease, and death usually occurs before age ten.

Duchenne Muscular Dystrophy

This is an X-linked genetic disorder associated with progressive muscle weakness beginning at about three or four years of age. Affected boys eventually become unable to walk. Death usually occurs as a result of cardiac failure or respiratory infection by age twenty.

Duchenne muscular dystrophy (DMD) is named after the French neurologist who first described it in 1861. Like other muscular dystrophies, DMD is inherited — it is a genetic condition. It is transmitted by an altered gene on the X chromosome in an X-linked recessive pattern, the same pattern that is seen in hemophilia and color blindness. Only males are affected. Females, who rarely show any symptoms, may be carriers of the defective gene and can pass on the disease to their sons and, indirectly, to their grandsons through daughters who are carriers. One other type of muscular dystrophy — Becker muscular dystrophy — is also X-linked. It is similar to DMD but has later onset and is considerably less severe.

The mother of a boy with DMD may not be a carrier. The DMD gene she transmits may have become defective as the result of a spontaneous change in the particular egg cell that joined with a sperm cell to develop into the child. Such a change in a gene is known as a new mutation and is a possibility to be considered when DMD occurs in families where there is no previous history of the disease. Nevertheless, absence of a family history does not mean that a case of DMD has resulted from a new mutation. It may be that the mutation has been in the family for a number of generations and has not shown up before, just by chance; or the mutation may have occurred in a family member only one or two generations earlier. In any event, the mother of a child who is the only family member with DMD may or may not be a carrier. It is a major goal of genetic evaluation to determine whether or not she is.

Retinitis Pigmentosa

Scientists recently isolated the gene responsible for retinoblastoma (an inherited form of eye cancer that affects the retina, the site of visual receptors in the eye). Normal persons have two copies of the retinoblas-toma gene. The protein product of the gene appears to protect cells in the eye against unregulated growth. Children with a hereditary suscep-tibility to retinoblastoma have just one copy, and inactivation of the single copy by environmental or other factors leads to eye cancer.

Cooley's Anemia

A fatal blood disorder peculiar to people of Mediterranean origin, this is also called Mediterranean anemia and thalassemia. Thalassemia trait occurs when a person inherits *one* thalassemia gene from only one parent. A person with the thalassemia trait is usually unaware that he or she has the condition. If one parent has the thalassemia trait and the other parent does *not*, there is a 50-percent chance (one-in-two chance) with *each* pregnancy that the baby will be born with the thalassemia trait.

Thalassemia *major* occurs when a person inherits two thalassemia genes, one from each parent. Known as Cooley's anemia in this form, it is a severe and eventually fatal blood disorder. If both parents have the thalassemia trait, there is a 25-percent chance (one-in-four chance) with *each* pregnancy that the baby will have thalassemia major.

People with the thalassemia trait are less likely to die from malaria, if they catch it, than other people. In the past, in countries where malaria was very common, people with the thalassemia trait survived malaria when other people died. They passed the trait on to their children. Malaria used to occur in many countries, all of which now have quite a large number of people with the thalassemia trait. For instance, in Cyprus one in seven people have the trait (both Turkish and Greek Cypriots), and in Greece one in twelve people have it. In Italy and all of the Middle East and Asia, including India, Pakistan, Hong Kong and Vietnam, the number of people with the thalassemia trait varies from one in fifty to one in ten from one area to another. In Africa and the West Indies about one in fifty people have the trait, whereas about one in every thousand people of British origin have it.

Children with thalassemia major are normal at birth but become anemic between the ages of three months and eighteen months. They become pale, do not sleep well, do not want to eat, and may vomit their food. If children with this disorder are not treated, they have miserable lives and usually die at between one and eight years of age.

More than two million Americans of Mediterranean heritage are carriers of the genetic trait for Cooley's anemia. If you have the thalassemia trait, but your partner has normal blood, there is no chance that your children will inherit thalassemia major, though they may have the thalassemia trait. If both you and your partner have the trait, then, again in *each* pregnancy there is a one-in-four chance that you will have a child with thalassemia major.

If you are at risk, your physician can discuss the options available to you. There is a simple and accurate test for thalassemia that requires a sample of blood taken from a vein. However, the test is not done routinely and must be requested by name.

Alcoholism

Alcoholism is strongly familial. It runs through many generations and there are some remarkable pedigrees. The past twenty years have witnessed several important advances in our search for knowledge about genetic and other family linkages to alcoholism and alcohol abuse, among them the recognition that family members of alcoholics clearly are at increased risk of alcoholism.

The observation that alcoholism runs in families is not new; references to this phenomenon appear in the Bible and in classical Greek and Roman literature, but recent research has provided evidence that points persuasively to heredity's role in the development of the disease. However, while research shows an increased risk among people who have alcoholism in their families, it also shows that not everyone with this inherited vulnerability develops the disease, not all alcoholics have a familial history of the disease, and only a minority of those with alcoholic family members actually develop the disease.

Evidence for genetic predisposition to alcoholism continues to grow. It is now widely accepted by researchers in the field that alcoholism results from the interaction of heredity and environment. Support for this conclusion comes from a variety of studies of familial alcoholism, from studies of twins and of adoptees separated from their biological parents at an early age, and from animal breeding experiments.

Studies of adoptees in Sweden have identified two types of genetic predisposition to alcoholism: milieu-limited and male-limited. The former susceptibility occurs in both sexes and requires environmental stimulation to become expressed as alcoholism; the latter, transmitted only by the biological fathers of the adoptees, is highly heritable and gives rise to severe early-onset alcoholism often requiring extensive treatment. It should be noted that these predispositions were identified by studying data from official records, not by conducting clinical examinations.

Researchers are also making progress in identifying biochemical markers of genetic predisposition to alcoholism and its associated disorders. Much of the work is centered on genetic variation in alcohol-metabolizing enzymes, especially on how such genetic variations could affect tissue levels of acetaldehyde, the first metabolic product of alcohol. Elevated acetaldehyde levels have been implicated as the cause of the dysphoric or uncomfortable alcohol flush reaction that is common in Orientals. It is hypothesized that higher acetaldehyde, and the uncomfortable flushing reaction it can cause, provides protection against excessive drinking and that this may account for lower alcoholism rates among Orientals.

Another potential biochemical marker of genetic susceptibility to alcoholism is low levels of platelet monoamine oxidase. Studies have shown that alcoholics and their nonalcoholic children both tend to have lower levels of this enzyme. Indications are that low monoamine oxidase levels are a genetic marker of susceptibility to male-limited alcoholism, and that monoamineoxidase assay — testing for these levels — may allow early identification of at-risk individuals. If these findings can be replicated, the implications for prevention and treatment are significant.

Polycystic Kidney Disease (PKD)

Polycystic kidney disease, called PKD, is an inherited disease which causes cysts in both kidneys. It may often cause cysts or outpouchings in the liver, pancreas, colon and blood vessels in the brain, and perhaps affect the heart valves, too. It appears to occur throughout the world, with the latest data showing some 320,000 to 400,000 cases in the United States.

You get PKD from a parent who has the disease. If you are in a family that has the disease, but your parents are not affected, you will not get it. If one of your parents has PKD you have a fifty-fifty chance of contracting it. If you are in a family that has the disease, but you do not have it, you cannot pass it on to your children. PKD is an autosomal dominant type disease and is a major cause of kidney failure.

Alzheimer's Disease

Alzheimer's disease is the fourth-leading cause of death in the United States. However, recent research indicates only 10 percent of cases are clearly inherited. For the present, only people with Alzheimer's in their family history can be tested.

Manic Depression

A marker for inherited manic depression has been discovered recently. This mood-swing disorder strikes about one to two million American adults. In this case, the gene is thought to predispose to mood disorders rather than to always cause the disease, with environmental influences believed to trigger this inherited tendency into full-blown manic depression. (See chapter 4 for a discussion of genetics and mental illness.)

Malignant Hyperthermia

Malignant hyperthermia or MH is called the anesthesiologist's nightmare because the sudden, unexpected death of a healthy child or young adult undergoing minor surgery is a tragedy almost beyond comprehension in this day of modern medical miracles. Yet perhaps one in two hundred persons may be at risk of developing the deadly MH syndrome. Of those who develop it, up to 20 percent may die. Some who survive will be left with severe brain damage, failed kidneys, or impaired function of other major organs.

MH is a chain reaction of symptoms (a syndrome) triggered in previously unidentified individuals by commonly used general anesthetics and some other drugs. The syndrome is characterized by greatly increased body metabolism, muscle rigidity, and fever to 110 degrees or more.

The basis for the underlying problem in some families is a single defective gene, usually inherited from one parent. In other families, according to the Malignant Hyperthermia Association of the United States (MHAUS), the genetic pattern is not clear.

Although other patterns of inheritance have not been ruled out, most families appear to have passed the MH gene along in an autosomal dominant mode. Both sexes can therefore suffer from the disorder and transmit the gene to sons and daughters, and the abnormal gene will express itself even when its partner gene is normal. So if one parent is normal for this gene and the other is affected, each of their children has a 50-percent chance of receiving the normal gene and a 50-percent chance of receiving the abnormal gene.

The patterns of inheritance have become apparent in a few large families where several MH deaths have occurred in successive generations, or from families where several people have undergone muscle biopsy testing. Not everyone who has the MH gene develops an MH episode during every anesthetic. Identification of inheritance patterns in families has been hampered by the cumbersome nature of diagnostic tests. When a simple and readily available test becomes available, the genetics of MH will be much clearer and better understood.

MH has been identified in almost every country in the Western world as well as in Japan, Australia and New Zealand. It has no racial boundaries, although in the United States it most often affects Caucasians of northern European heritage. Both sexes are equally at risk of MH, but it occurs more often in males than females.

According to MHAUS, there is no concrete scientific data, but some physical characteristics do appear frequently in MH-susceptible families.

While these characteristics cannot be used to diagnose MH, they are sometimes a helpful indication of possibly being at risk. These traits are:

- a history of unexplained high fevers
- unusual muscle weakness
- an inability to exercise in high temperatures
- eye muscle abnormalities, such as droopy eyelids, crossed eyes or wandering eyes
- spinal deformities such as scoliosis (an abnormal lateral or sideward curve to the spine) or pigeon breast
- a life-long history of muscle cramps, particularly when unrelated to activity
- joint abnormalities such as frequent partial dislocations, clubfoot, etc.

Additionally, male children who fit a certain rare set of physical criteria known as the King-Denborough Syndrome seem to be at particular risk of developing MH. These children are usually short, have a pigeon breast and distinctive facial features including high forehead, low-set ears and a downward slant to the eyes.

Hereditary Ataxia

Hereditary ataxia refers to a special group of inherited spinocerebellar (brain and spinal cord) degenerations. It respects no particular age or race. The gene(s) responsible for ataxia (literally, "without order or incoordination") are thought to cause the production of an abnormal protein. This causes degeneration of the nerve cells, which reduces nerve signals to the muscles. The cells affected are primarily in the brain (cerebellum) and spinal cord. As the nerve cells continue to degenerate, muscles become less and less responsive to commands from the brain, causing coordination problems to become more pronounced.

Hereditary ataxia is diagnosed from a person's medical and family history and a complete neurological evaluation. At this time it cannot be diagnosed before symptoms appear, and currently there are no specific blood tests or other tests to indicate ataxia. There is no prenatal test to determine if an unborn child has inherited the ataxia gene.

Dominant ataxia, sometimes referred to as Marie atrophe or Olivopontocerebellar atrophe (OPCA), is passed on as a dominant hereditary disease. Each child born of a parent with dominant ataxia has a fifty-fifty chance of getting ataxia. If a child does not develop ataxia, his or her children in turn cannot become afflicted and future generations are free of the disease. The symptoms usually appear around ages twenty to forty.

However, in recessive hereditary ataxia parents do not exhibit symptoms, but they each carry a recessive gene which may cause ataxia in their offspring. The genetic path of recessive ataxia is impossible to predict. The recessive gene may lie dormant for generations until two people with the defective gene have children. Each child of recessive ataxia parents has the following genetic odds: a 25-percent chance of being free, a 50-percent chance of being a carrier without showing symptoms, and a 25-percent chance of having the disease.

One of the most common recessive ataxias is Friedreich's ataxia, which usually begins in the childhood or teenage years. While it is thought that many of the inherited ataxias have onset early in the life span, there now appears to be good evidence that there are forms of hereditary ataxia which have onset in the age range of fifty to sixty-five years. These may be inherited in either a dominant or a recessive pattern, depending on family history.

The aim of a recent research project has been to detect a genetic marker that is linked to the gene for Friedreich's ataxia (FRDA) so it can be used to determine more precisely the probability that an individual is a carrier of this recessively inherited disease. The families participating in this study are those of Acadian ancestry in southwestern Louisiana with at least one member who has Friedreich's ataxia. In 1985 and 1986 field trips were made to various parts of southwestern Louisiana to collect blood samples from members of these families. It was found that all of the obligate carriers of the gene for FRDA (that is, parents of affected individuals) in these seventeen families are related to one another, usually as fourth, fifth and sixth cousins, although with many different lines of descent. When possible, blood samples were collected from the grandparents of the affected individuals and all other first-degree relatives of the obligate carriers, and the research continues.

Arthritis

Chances are you or someone you know or some of your ancestors have had arthritis, since it affects about 37 million Americans, or one in every three families. Some of the most common types of arthritis and its associated diseases are rheumatoid arthritis, osteoarthritis, systemic lupus erythematosus, scleroderma, and gout; others are juvenile arthritis, ankylosing spondylitis, psoriatic arthritis, infectious arthritis, fibrositis, bursitis and tendinitis.

Scientists have known for about fifteen years that people with certain genetic traits, or markers, are more likely than others to develop certain types of arthritis. For example, the genetic marker called HLA-B27 is present in almost all people with ankylosing spondylitis, a form of arthritis that affects the spine. However, about 7 percent of perfectly healthy people also have the same marker, so it alone cannot cause the disease.

Likewise, a group of genes known as HLA-DR4 is associated with rheumatoid arthritis (see below), and scientists are currently working to identify the exact gene or genes implicated in that disease. Similar research is going on to find the specific genes involved in systemic lupus erythematosus, an arthritis-related disease that can have wide-ranging effects on the skin, kidneys, joints and other tissues. However, genes are not the whole story in arthritis. That is, the arthritis-related diseases are not straightforward inherited disorders like hemophilia or sickle-cell anemia. Popular among scientists is the "trigger" theory, which says that different viruses or bacteria may be needed to set the disease in motion in people born with the susceptibility. This means that given the conditions of the "wrong" gene types and the "wrong" virus or bacteria, an abnormal immune response may be triggered, resulting in a wide range of misdirected immune reactions, which eventually lead to chronic pain and tissue destruction.

"One of the big areas of study in future years will be genetics," predicts Dr. Frederick McDuffie, medical director for the Arthritis Foundation.

"From our current studies, we already know that some arthritis-related diseases probably result from the interaction of genes with each other or with environmental agents such as drugs, viruses or bacteria. Scientists are now trying to discover exactly how genes influence the development of these diseases."

Rheumatoid Arthritis — It is believed that there may be an unknown agent that causes rheumatoid arthritis, but only in people with a genetic, or inherited, tendency toward the disease. One clue supporting this concept is that most people with rheumatoid arthritis have the genetic marker HLA-DR4, a tissue type occurring in about one-fourth of the population. However, most people with the HLA-DR4 type will not get rheumatoid arthritis. Those who have it simply may develop the disease more readily.

Osteoarthritis — This is the oldest and most common disease of mankind. Almost 16 million Americans have this disease. It is also called degenerative joint disease, arthrosis or hypertrophic arthritis. For years, osteoarthritis has been considered a result of normal wear and tear of the body over the course of a person's lifetime. However, many researchers today think there are probably several factors leading to osteoarthritis. A genetic or inherited factor may be one.

A fairly common complication of osteoarthritis is the presence of bony growths in the finger joints. If they occur in the end joints of the fingers, they are called Heberden's nodes. Heberden's nodes appear most often in women with osteoarthritis and sometimes occur as early as age forty. They tend to run in families, according to the Arthritis Foundation.

Tay-Sachs and Allied Diseases

Tay-Sachs disease (TSD) is a fatal genetic disorder in children that causes the progressive destruction of the central nervous system. This destructive process begins in the fetus early in pregnancy, although the disease is not clinically apparent until the child is several months old. By the time a child with TSD is four or five years old, the nervous system is so badly affected that life itself cannot be supported. Even with the best of care, TSD children die by the age of five.

Tay-Sachs disease is named for Warren Tay (1843-1927), a British ophthalmologist, who described a case in 1881 that was characterized by a cherry-red spot on the retina of the eye, and for Bernard Sachs, a New York neurologist, whose work several years later provided the first descriptions of the cellular changes in Tay-Sachs disease. Sachs, who observed many more cases, recognized the familial nature of the disorder and pointed out that most Tay-Sachs babies were of Eastern European Jewish origin.

TSD is one of a group of about thirty genetic disorders called storage diseases. These disorders share a common biochemical defect: the inability to break down and dispose of waste products in the cells.

TSD is transmitted as an autosomal recessive disorder; that is, it is transmitted through the genes in the same way as hair color and eye color are passed from parent to child. Both parents must be carriers of the recessive TSD gene in order to produce a Tay-Sachs baby. Carrier status does not affect the mother and father physically in any way, since a person who is a carrier can transmit a particular genetic trait to an offspring but is not ill with the disease. If only one parent is a TSD carrier, there is no chance of producing a TSD baby.

High-risk couples, in which both the man and the woman are carriers, have a 25-percent chance with *each* pregnancy of producing a child with Tay-Sachs disease. The child must inherit the inactive TSD gene from each parent to have the disease. There is a 50-percent chance, again with *each* pregnancy, of producing a child who is a carrier like the parent, and a 25-percent chance that the child will be neither a carrier nor be affected.

Recessive genetic diseases like Tay-Sachs often occur more frequently, though not exclusively, in a defined population. A person's chances of being a TSD carrier are greatest if he or she is of Eastern European (Ashkenazi) Jewish descent. Approximately one in every twenty-five Jews in the United States is a carrier of the TSD gene; in the general population, the carrier rate is one in 250. Approximately 85 percent of the children affected with TSD are Jewish. However, Tay-Sachs can and does occur in Jews of Sephardic origin and in the non-Jewish community. There is a noticeable incidence of TSD in non-Jewish French-Canadians living near the St. Lawrence River, for example.

The TSD gene can be carried without being expressed through many generations. It is conceivable that it might *never* surface. Since 1971 prenatal testing has been coupled with intensive educational campaigns among Jewish populations to provide voluntary mass screening of adults in an effort to identify carriers. Couples planning their families, alerted by the publicity about Tay-Sachs disease, its cause and prevention, have blood samples taken at Tay-Sachs prevention centers in hospitals or at public screenings conducted in conjunction with qualified medical personnel. While testing is aimed at couples of child-bearing age, it is desirable to screen as many of the target population as possible. Very often a couple who have completed their family will want to know if any of their children could be carriers. If such a couple is tested and learns that neither the husband nor the wife is a carrier, they can assure all their children that they are not carriers. However, should one or both be found to be carriers, they know it will be imperative for their children and other family members to be tested.

Niemann-Pick Disease — In 1914, Albert Niemann, a German pediatrician, described a young Jewish child with an enlarged liver and spleen, enlarged lymph glands, swelling and a darkening of the skin of the face. The child had brain and nervous system impairment and died in less than six months, before the age of two. Later, in the 1920s, Ludwig Pick studied tissues of such children after they had died and provided the evidence that they were victims of a different and distinct disorder from Tay-Sachs and diseases of that type.

Actually, Niemann-Pick disease affects people of all ethnic origins, but the majority of the infants who contract it, as with Tay-Sachs, are of Ashkenazi Jewish ancestry. As with Tay-Sachs, Niemann-Pick is an inherited disease that is caused by a recessive gene. The gene may affect either males or females and Niemann-Pick is therefore referred to as an autosomal recessive gene disorder. Families at risk have the same one-in-four probability of an affected child with each pregnancy as in Tay-Sachs disease.

It is particularly important to use precise and accurate biochemical tests with this disease, as with other storage disorders, since the features of several of these diseases tend to resemble one another to some extent. Therefore, especially when anticipating a pregnancy within a family suspected of a history of Niemann-Pick disease, or Tay-Sachs, it is essential to have tests done on persons at risk — at centers qualified to conduct these tests.

Sandhoff's Disease — The inheritance of the Sandhoff gene is exactly the same as it is for the Tay-Sachs gene, and the disease is similar to Tay-Sachs.

Gaucher's Disease — A disease originally described in 1882 by Phillipe Gaucher, a French physician, many investigators have since refined our understanding of this disease. In the early 1900s, American physicians were the first to recognize its familial transmission. It is an autosomal recessive genetic disorder, with the same pattern of inheritance as Tay-Sachs.

The three subtypes of Gaucher's disease are distinguished by their clinical severity and course, and by the presence or absence of neurologic complications. Type I is the most common and does not have mental or neurologic involvement. This disease is found primarily in Jewish individuals of Central and Eastern European ancestry. Type II is extremely rare and its occurrence is not linked to any particular ethnic or demographic group. Type III begins in early childhood, has mild to severe neurologic involvement, and is very rare except in Sweden, where most patients have been found.

Each of the three types of Gaucher's disease is genetically distinct and "breeds true" in affected families — that is, no two types of Gaucher's disease occur in the same family. All three types of Gaucher's disease are inherited "storage" diseases. It was discovered in 1965 that they result from the deficiency of an enzyme called acid B-glucosidase, which is necessary for the breakdown of a particular fatty substance, glucosyl ceramide. This substance is normally present in very small amounts in all body cells, but in patients with Gaucher's disease, glucosyl ceramide becomes abnormally stored, primarily in unique cells called Gaucher's cells.

Type I usually becomes apparent in childhood or early adulthood, when patients initially show an enlarged spleen or develop hematologic or orthopedic problems. It is not exclusive to individuals of Ashkenazi Jewish ancestry, but it is estimated that one in every twenty-five Jewish individuals of Central and Eastern European ancestry is a carrier of the Gaucher's Type I gene and that one in every 2,500 Ashkenazi Jews is afflicted with this disease. Gaucher's disease is therefore the most common genetic disease in the Ashkenazi Jewish population. Concerned couples and individuals can be tested for the Type I Gaucher's gene.

Krabbe's Disease — Although this disease occurs in all ethnic groups, it is most common in the Scandinavian countries. The disease was first described in 1916 by a Scandinavian neurologist-pathologist named Knud H. Krabbe. The disorder belongs to the same general category of genetic lipid storage diseases as Tay-Sachs disease, Sandhoff's disease, Niemann-Pick disease and Gaucher's disease. Krabbe's disease is unusual in many respects. Patients appear normal at birth, but parents usually notice the first signs of the condition in their children at four to six months, when the baby becomes sensitive and irritable in response to noise, touch, and strong light and begins to cry frequently without apparent cause. Development slows down and then, rapidly, progressive mental and motor deterioration set in.

Unlike Tay-Sachs or Sandhoff's, in which nerve cells are the target of the disease, Krabbe's disease affects mainly the white matter of the brain — so named because the nerve fibers passing through this region are covered by white myelin. The disease is inherited as a recessive trait; therefore, both parents must be carriers of the abnormal gene for them to have affected babies.

Two lysosomal storage diseases that do not follow the recessive pattern are Fabry's disease and Hunter's syndrome (see above). These two are sex-linked, or X-linked, disorders. Only male children are affected.

Consanguinity

While marriages among first cousins are fairly rare in American families today, you may discover that in earlier generations your families did intermarry that closely. If your parents were first cousins you are at a higher risk than average for some genetic disorders. Lesser degrees of consanguinity than that of first cousins pose proportionately lower risks. For example, second cousins (that is, children of first cousins) have only 1/32 of their genes in common and third cousins share only one in 128. As far as recessive abnormalities are concerned, the only consanguinity that matters is the actual blood relationship of the parents — related marriages confined to the forebears of one partner alone are irrelevant. All that is important is the extent to which husband and wife tend to share the same genes, and this depends only upon their relationship to each other.

The great majority of affected persons are the offspring of parents who are normal to all outward appearances. There is a familial incidence; that is, sibships frequently occur in which more than one child is affected. Where an abnormality is rare, then there usually is an undue proportion of consanguineous marriages found among the parents of affected persons. The rarer the defect the higher the proportion of consanguineous marriages. Affected persons who marry normals have only normal offspring in the great majority of cases.

There are several populations in the world with very high rates of consanguineous marriage. In some parts of the Middle East the frequency of first-cousin marriages is 30 percent or higher, and high levels are also found, for example, among some populations in India and in the rural areas of Japan. In practical terms, a cousin marriage in a traditionally inbred community is less likely to result in children manifesting recessive disease. While a tradition of cousin marriage does not, in the long run, lead to a high frequency of severe recessive disease, when such affected children do occur, their parents are still blood relatives more often than would be expected from the general rate of consanguinity in the population. For example, for a defect with a frequency as high as one in 10,000 and a rate of cousin marriage of 25 percent, about 67 percent of the parents of affected children would be first cousins.

Since so many genetic disorders occur in particular ethnic groups or in families that have intermarried, the ethnic background of your ancestors and any consanguineous marriages are important items to include in your family history.

4 — Your Mental and Behavioral Roots

esearch groups are hot on the trail of genetic markers for certain panic disorders that occur even without stress. Encouraged by the discovery of genetic markers for dyslexia, Alzheimer's and manic depression, many geneticists now are being drawn to the study of mental and behavioral disturbances.

But what does all of this research mean to you and your family? Well, if you knew you had a susceptibility to alcoholism or that your adopted child does, you probably would never take that first drink. And you would do everything in your power to educate your children about its risk to them.

Researchers at the University of British Columbia in Vancouver have reported finding a possible genetic marker for schizophrenia. Until the 1960s scientists believed that environment alone caused schizophrenia. However, many people, especially genealogists, figured that schizophrenia ran in families. They just reasoned that crazy mothers doing crazy things turned out crazy kids. It was common sense. But the astounding thing that has been learned is that kids are just as likely to become schizophrenic if their mothers give them up for adoption and never see them again. The key to unlocking the secrets of schizophrenia will probably come when it is learned how environment and heredity work together.

Huntington's disease and Alzheimer's disease are two neurological disorders that strike late in life. Huntington's disease is always caused by a gene, but only 10 percent of Alzheimer's cases have been clearly traced to heredity, according to James Gussella, director of the Neurogenetics Laboratory at Massachusetts General Hospital in Boston, who was part of a team that discovered genetic markers for these two diseases. He believes that tests for predisposition to Alzheimer's will be limited to families with a history of the disease. When heredity plays a role, the disease is more likely to strike in the late forties and fifties than after age sixty, when the majority of cases occur.

It is difficult to spot the early warning signs of mental disease because there may be a multitude of biochemical abnormalities involved. In one Pennsylvania Amish family with a history of manic depression, for example, the culprit gene was traced to chromosome 11. By contrast, a gene on the female sex chromosome, or X chromosome, is thought to account for the same disorder in a large Jewish family in Israel. Researchers believe studies of other ethnic groups may turn up yet more genes for manic depression.

Environmental factors usually figure prominently in any mental disturbance. However, genetic markers have proved to be powerful predictors — at least in the Amish and Jewish families referred to above. In both cases 75 to 80 percent of individuals with the familial markers had at least one episode of manic depression.

Early diagnosis offers the possibility of early intervention. Advances in the field will eventually permit preschoolers to be screened for different forms of the reading disability known as dyslexia. That way remedial training can begin at a young age, when it makes an enormous difference, says Dr. Herbert Lubs, a University of Miami geneticist who uncovered a marker for the disability. "And you avoid all the psychological problems that arise when a child is labeled retarded or a low achiever."

Is Mental Illness Inherited?

Researchers recently have found, by using the tools of molecular biology along with the handwritten genealogical records of Amish families, that the mental disorder known as manic depression is indeed at least partly a matter of bloodlines. In a report published in the journal *Nature* they conclusively linked cases of manic depression in an Amish family to genes in a specific region of human chromosome 11.

"This is the first demonstration of a possible genetic basis for one of the major mental disorders," says Dr. Darrel Regier, director of the division of clinical research at the National Institute of Mental Health (NIMH). "The study ushers in a new era of psychiatric research."

Usually beginning somewhere between the ages of fifteen and thirty-five, manic depression afflicts about one in every hundred people. Researchers have long suspected that heredity plays a role in some if not all cases, and the Amish presented an ideal setting in which to test that hypothesis. The Amish have large families (seven children on the average) and keep outstanding genealogical records. Best of all, they represent a closed genetic pool. All 12,500 Amish in Lancaster County, Pennsylvania are descended from twenty or thirty couples who emigrated from Europe in the early 1700s, with only a handful of outsiders ever having married into this group.

Though manic depression is no more common among the Amish than other groups, research turned up thirty-two active cases. All proved to have family histories of the disease going back several generations. Curiously, all of the twenty-six suicides documented in the community since 1880 occurred in just four of these families.

The study focused on three families, spread through three generations — an 81-member clan. Fourteen members had been diagnosed as having manic depression and another five as having other mental disorders. The researchers were also able to confirm that children of individuals with this marked abnormality have a 50-percent chance of inheriting it. However, only 63 percent of those carrying the gene show signs of the disorder. This suggests that other factors — perhaps environment — also play a role in bringing on the disease. The decade-long study yielded the first evidence that there is a gene somewhere along the tip of a specific chromosome that predisposes its bearers to manic depression, and possibly to severe depression without mania.

The same genetic defect does not play a role in all manic depression, however. Two other studies revealed no link between the chromosome 11 site and manic depression in six non-Amish families prone to the disease. However, these findings do not undermine the important discovery of a genetic basis for the ailment. Sevilla Detera-Wadleigh, a psychiatrist who led one of the other studies, suggests that more than one gene may be involved in manic depression.

Scientists now are trying to identify the particular gene or genes responsible for manic depression. This will enable them to understand the biochemical basis for the disease, which could lead to better treatment. (Presently the drug lithium carbonate is effective in 70 to 75 percent of cases.) It could also lead to tests for the diagnosis and identification of people at risk.

Alcoholism, Personality and Your Genes

Alcoholism shows up in people of diverse personalities and economic backgrounds, and in all ethnic groups. There are the alcoholic skid-row bums, wealthy congressmen, bored housewives, talented high school students and famous entertainers, as well as your co-workers, neighbors and loved ones. Some are happy-go-lucky tipplers; others are raving drunk maniacs. This has stymied researchers in their efforts to understand the underlying biological or psychological factors that lead to alcoholism. Now some researchers think there may be at least one definable segment of the alcoholic population — those with the character disorder called antisocial personality (ASP).

Antisocial personalities (previously labeled sociopaths) tend to be charming, manipulative, attention-seeking, rebellious, impulsive, egocentric, and ready abusers of drugs, other people and themselves. Antisocial personalities make up perhaps 25 percent of the total alcoholic population. This is an extraordinary ratio because the prevalence of ASP in the general population is only about 3 percent.

ASP may prove to be a key in the search for genetic markers for alcoholism, according to psychologist Ralph Tarter of the University of Pittsburgh. The traits typical of ASP, he contends, may be a "behavioral manifestation of a genetic vulnerability" to both alcoholism and ASP. "In other words," he says, "some people inherit a behavioral propensity that heightens their risk for becoming sociopathic or alcoholic."

The observation that alcoholism tends to run in families is a very old one, but until recently lack of appropriate studies has made it impossible to know whether this familial clustering is due to heredity, environment, or perhaps both. Recent research, according to the National Institute on

Alcohol Abuse and Alcoholism, has provided evidence that both heredity and environment are involved in the genesis of many cases of alcoholism.

Several studies have shown that sons of alcoholics are many times more likely to become alcoholic than are the sons of nonalcoholics. Some early studies suggest that genetic transmission of one or more biological characteristics may predispose the sons of alcoholics to alcoholism. An inherited predisposition to alcoholism has also been found in women and is evidently transmitted through the mother.

A study in Denmark of 5,483 persons who had been adopted at an early age revealed that the sons of alcoholics who had been adopted by other families were more than three times as likely to become alcoholic as the adopted sons of nonalcoholics. These findings were later confirmed in a study of 2,324 adoptees in Sweden. In the Swedish study, male adoptees whose biological fathers were severely alcoholic had a 20-percent incidence of alcohol abuse, compared with 6 percent in the adopted sons of nonalcoholics. Male adoptees whose biological mothers were alcohol abusers had a 33-percent incidence of alcohol abuse compared with 19 percent in the control group.

These adoption studies strongly support the hypothesis that genetics contributes to susceptibility to alcoholism. The alcoholic adoptees had been separated from their biological parents before the age of three years and in most cases during the first few months of life, and thus removed from any predisposing environmental influences arising from an alcoholic home. The predominant environmental influence therefore came from their adoptive homes, not from the stressful home life that might be associated with parental alcoholism. Nevertheless, in both studies sons adopted from alcoholics had about a threefold greater chance of becoming alcohol abusers or alcoholics.

An effect of parental alcoholism was also found in adopted women. Daughters adopted from alcoholic mothers had more than three times the frequency of alcohol abuse than the daughters adopted from nonalcoholic parents: 10.8 percent of the daughters of alcoholic biological mothers were alcohol abusers compared with 2.8 percent of daughters who did not have an alcoholic biological parent.

The evidence from such studies is compelling: biological inheritance can be a major factor in the development of alcohol abuse and alcoholism. Furthermore, these studies reveal the existence of two forms of inherited predisposition — one that is strongly influenced by postnatal environment, and one in which the development of alcoholism is strongly influenced by the sex of the individual.

The Swedish adoption studies revealed the existence of two types of genetic predisposition to alcoholism:

- The more common type, called milieu-limited (or Type I) alcoholism, accounts for most cases of alcoholism. It occurs in both men and women, is usually not severe, and is associated with mild, untreated, adult-onset alcohol abuse in either biological parent.

- The other type is called male-limited (or Type II) alcoholism. This severe type of predisposition is found only in men, and accounts for about 25 percent of all male alcoholics in the general population. Its transmission appears to be unaffected by the environment. In families with male-limited susceptibility, alcohol abuse was nine times more frequent in the adopted sons regardless of their postnatal environment. Interestingly, male-limited susceptibility was associated with severe alcoholism in the biological father but not with alcohol abuse in the biological mother. Male-limited alcoholism frequently developed in the biological fathers when they were adolescents.

While no evidence was found that men with male-limited alcoholism can transmit the same susceptibility to their daughters, it was discovered that in adopted women whose biological fathers had this form of hereditary alcoholism there was a greater frequency of diversiform somatization — a psychosomatic condition characterized by frequent complaints of pain or discomfort, usually medically unexplained, in various parts of the body. This suggests that women may inherit the same genetic factors that lead to male-limited alcoholism but express those factors in different ways.

Experts caution, however, that it is erroneous to conclude that every alcoholic or alcohol abuser harbors a genetic predisposition to alcoholism. Numerous alcoholics do not have alcoholic first-degree (close) relatives, and it still may be that many cases of alcoholism arise from psychological, social, and cultural causes, not genetic ones. A fatalistic attitude about alcoholism is not warranted by these studies either. Sporadic, nonfamilial alcoholism is preventable and treatable. So is milieu-limited alcoholism, and although it may be difficult to treat, its effects can at least be mitigated.

Alcoholics who have a family history of alcoholism, and therefore a possible genetic basis for their disease, should not despair but should keep in mind that other diseases also have a genetic component. It is known, for example, that genetics play a major role in diabetes, yet diabetics can be helped, especially when they take responsibility for their own recovery. The same is true of alcoholics.

Current Research — A recent adoption study in Iowa confirmed that the greatest single predictor of alcoholism in a son is alcoholism in a father. Statistics show that 25 percent of the sons of alcoholic fathers are alcoholic, while 10 percent of the general population in America is alcoholic. Familial alcoholism, which means a person has a close relative who is alcoholic, afflicts about half the alcoholic population.

Researchers are now focusing on the families of alcoholics, particularly on the population most susceptible to the disease — young sons of alcoholics — in an attempt to pinpoint biological indicators of vulnerability. Some scientists are looking for differences in alcohol metabolism and blood chemistry, and there is also increasing interest in brain function. Examinations of those who are especially vulnerable to the disease, for example, have shown that some changes in cognitive and motor function, formerly attributed to alcoholism, take place in some people *before* the onset of the disease.

A number of electroencephalogram (EEG) studies have found differences between the brain waves of alcoholics and nonalcoholics as well as between the children of alcoholics and of nonalcoholics. Meanwhile, other researchers have been finding indirect evidence for neurological deficits in high-risk subjects (the sons of alcoholic parents). This evidence comes from neuropsychological studies that attempt to infer deficits in brain functions through tests of motor and spatial abilities and problem-solving. Psychologist Oscar Parsons, of the University of Oklahoma, examined four types of drinkers: familial alcoholics, nonfamilial alcoholics, and social drinkers with and without family histories of alcoholism. He tested them for verbal abilities, learning and memory, and abstracting, problem-solving and perceptual-motor skills. The alcoholics performed more poorly than did the social drinkers on *all* the tests. Within these two groups, those with a family history of alcoholism performed worse than did those without. The difference was especially striking in the more complex problem-solving tests and the perceptual-motor tests. Parsons concludes that familial alcoholism has an independent effect on test performance, and that it probably deserves to be regarded as "a distinct subcategory of alcoholism."

The finding that many persons who seem to be genetically predisposed to alcoholism have mild neurological deficits does not explain why they should be particularly vulnerable to compulsive and ultimately addictive drinking, though. Researchers do not yet know whether there are neurological defects linked to chemical abnormalities that generate alcohol craving, or whether there are particular emotional or behavioral problems that lead to compulsive drinking. One researcher, Thomas Babor, a social psychologist at the University of Connecticut, found that 40 percent of the people he studied in alcoholism clinics were antisocial personalities and that the two major precursors of alcoholism were family history and ASP. Furthermore, those with ASP had more alcoholism among their relatives and had a more severe form of the disease. They started earlier, drank more and sought help at an earlier age (thirty-three), on the average, than did the other alcoholics, who didn't seek help on average until the age of thirty-nine.

What makes the correlation between ASP and alcoholism significant in studying the genetics of alcoholism is that there appears to be a component of heritability to ASP. Additional support for a possible genetic link between ASP and alcoholism is provided by the fact that certain childhood disorders often precede the development of both ASP and alcoholism. One is attention deficit disorder, a catch-all diagnosis for traits including short attention span, impulsivity and hyperactivity. The other is childhood conduct disorder. Several studies have shown that severe alcoholics are more likely than nonalcoholics to have childhood histories marked by these symptoms.

As the evidence for a genetic component becomes stronger, researchers may take another look at long-term studies that show a preponderance of certain personality traits among alcoholics. Depression, for example, is a very common early psychopathology for female alcoholics.

The families of alcoholics are another major area of interest as researchers look for biological and behavioral clues to alcoholic susceptibility. Behavioral, biochemical and genetic researchers may eventually arrive at a "biobehavioral" explanation of alcoholism. Increasing recognition of the many facets of alcoholism is spurring more innovative approaches to prevention and more individually tailored treatment for this disease that occurs in so many families.

Behavior, Personality and Your Genes

"The genes you inherited from your parents play a major role in shaping your personality — who you are as a person," says behavior geneticist Robert Plomin. "Shyness shows the most evidence of genetic influence of any personality trait," he says.

Six or seven decades ago scientists believed that human behavior was largely a product of genetics, but in the period after World War II most psychologists tended to believe that babies arrived with a clean slate and that life experiences alone shaped a person's personality and behavior. However, by the late 1960s many behavioral scientists again began to think biology could influence behavior, but it wasn't until the 1970s that they started to talk about genetics again. Today, the research is concentrating on heredity.

In the late 1970s Dr. Plomin and his colleagues at the University of Colorado began studying shyness in children. The researchers compared the behavior of identical twins, who share 100 percent of their genes, and fraternal twins, who are no more alike genetically than ordinary brothers and sisters. Dr. Plomin found that identical twins behaved significantly more alike toward a stranger than did fraternal twins. He concluded that heredity clearly influences shyness.

In 1974 Dr. Plomin established the Colorado Adoption Project to study traits like intelligence, language ability and temperament, as well as shyness. Adoption creates a natural experiment because it separates the effects of children's genetic makeup from the environment in which they grow up. Today this is the largest study of its kind, with more than 250 adoptive families and 250 nonadoptive families still participating.

"Adoptive parents want to know how much a child will be like the biological parents and how much he'll be like the parents who raise him," Dr. Plomin says.

The Colorado Adoption Project confirmed that people inherit shyness. When adoptive mothers reported a shy child, the child's biological mother most likely was shy, too. It suggests that the genes that influence shyness in young kids continue to be active into adulthood. "Genes don't just have a one-shot influence at birth," according to Dr. Plomin.

By far the most powerful way to sort out genetic and environmental effects has been to combine studies of twins and adoptees. In Sweden (which keeps a registry of more than 25,000 pairs of twins born in that country) 750 pairs of adult twins, including more than 600 pairs of twins reared apart, were studied. These twins were asked about their lifestyle, personality, health and memories of childhood.

So far the study has found significant genetic influence on several aspects of personality, including shyness, emotionality, and activity level — the first time such an influence has been demonstrated in middle-age adults. One mind-boggling result, Dr. Plomin reports, was that identical twins reared *apart* report substantially similar perceptions about their home lives, even though they were raised in different homes. Plomin concludes that genes even influence perceptions and childhood memories. "Whether you see life through rose-colored glasses," he says, "seems to be a function of genetic dispositions."

Although behavior genetics is a long way from understanding what combinations of genes make some children shy, or emotional, or hyper-active, Dr. Plomin had some advice for parents in an article in *American Baby* (October 1987):

"We need to recognize that kids are different," he said. "It's not just what I as a parent did; they *came* that way. The second step is to respect those differences. That doesn't mean genes determine behavior and you can't change it. But it says that each child is an individual. We don't just mold our children like lumps of clay. We have to work *with* them to modify behavior."

Scientists have speculated for generations that people are the products of their genes, but proof was lacking. Now that has changed. Solid evidence demonstrates that our very characters are molded by heredity.

Scientists are turning up impressive evidence showing that heredity has a greater influence on personality and behavior than does upbringing.

"The pendulum is definitely swinging toward the side of the biologists and away from the environmentalists," says psychiatrist Herbert Leiderman of the Center for Advanced Study in the Behavioral Sciences at Stanford University.

Minnesota Twins Study

Much of the key investigative work on the role of genes in human behavior is done at the Minnesota Center for Twin and Adoption Research. Hundreds of sets of twins have been scrutinized and tested there since 1979. The center released its latest report late in 1986. After extensive testing of 348 sets of twins, including 44 pairs of identical twins raised separately, the institute's researchers concluded that how people think and act — their very personality — is determined more by genes than by society's influences. Even such things as respect for authority, a vivid imagination and a propensity to talk to strangers were found to be largely preordained at conception.

"The evidence is so compelling that it is hard to understand how people could *not* believe in the strong influence of genetics on behavior," says psychologist David Lykken of the Minnesota project.

Other studies have shown that genes seem to help explain alcoholism, depression and obesity — even sexual roles and preferences, and such phobias as fear of snakes and of strangers. The research bolsters what parents have always sensed: even within a single family, each child, right from birth, is different. While most parents think they are the primary molders of their child, they soon discover, usually with the arrival of the second one, that babies arrive in this world with built-in likes and dislikes. "Every parent of one child is an environmentalist, and every parent of more than one becomes a geneticist," says David Rowe, a University of Oklahoma psychologist who has studied how parents mold a child's character and ability.

The latest research clearly tips the scales toward the nature side of the nature-nurture debate. Researchers agree that people are creatures both of their genetic coding and of their cultural and environmental experience. All scientists are doing is learning the proportions of the recipe.

Work on personality traits that are determined by heredity rather than culture, based on new findings from the Minnesota Center for Twin and Adoption Research, shows some very close estimates of how much genes influence behavior in the general population. What the percentages will be in one individual is impossible to say, however.

The traits studied and analyzed, with the percentage of heredity given, are:

- Extroversion (mixes easily, is affable, likes to be the center of attention) — 61%

- Conformity (respects tradition and authority, follows the rules) — 60%

- Worry (is easily distressed and frustrated, feels vulnerable and sensitive) — 55%

- Creativity (tends to become lost in thought and abstraction) — 55%

- Paranoia (keeps to oneself, feels exploited, thinks "the world is out to get me") — 55%

- Optimism (is confident, cheerful and upbeat) — 54%

- Cautiousness (avoids risks and dangers, takes the safe route even if it is more difficult) — 51%

- Aggressiveness (tends to be physically violent, has a taste for revenge) — 48%

- Ambition (works hard at setting and achieving goals, is a perfectionist) — 46%

- Orderliness (plans carefully, tries to make rational decisions) — 43%

- Intimacy (prefers emotional closeness) — 33%

This project is considered the most comprehensive of its kind. The results of the tests in this study, which included forty-four pairs of identical twins who were brought up apart, were fascinating. Of the eleven key traits or clusters of traits analyzed in the study, researchers estimated that extroversion, conformity, vulnerability or resistance to stress, dedication to hard work and achievement, the capacity for being caught up in imaginative experiences, well-being, alienation, aggression and the shunning of risk or danger were all found to owe at least as much to nature as to nurture.

However, according to Thomas Bouchard, director of the study, the numbers so far may not be strictly accurate. "In general," he says, "the degree of genetic influence tends to be around 50 percent."

All the twins took several personality tests, answering more than 15,000 questions on subjects ranging from personal interests and values to phobias, aesthetic judgment and television and reading habits. Twins reared separately also took medical exams and intelligence tests and were queried on life history and stresses.

Since the early 1960s, several twin studies have reported that identical twins reared apart are actually more alike than those raised in the same home. For the Minnesota researchers and their allies, therefore, this study is just one more proof that parenting has its limits. "Parents should be blamed less for kids who have problems and take less credit for kids who turn out well," says twin researcher David Rowe.

"Roughly 40 percent of many personality differences between children can be accounted for by genetic inheritance," according to Robert Plomin. "There are three general dimensions of a child's personality that show substantial evidence of genetic influence," he says. "One is emotionality — how easily the child is aroused to joy or anger. Another is activity — the amount of general body movement and energy. A third is sociability — how much they like to be with people."

The environment provided by parents actually has very little influence on *broad* personality characteristics, notes Plomin. "Two adopted children from different biological parents who are reared in the same home," he reports, "essentially are no more similar in general personality to each other or to their parents than two children selected at random from different families."

While genes are usually cited as a reason why parents and children are similar to one another, they can also explain differences. "The first law of genetics," explains Dr. Plomin, "is that like begets like, and the second law is that like does not beget like. The reason is that children get half their genes from *each* parent. Since they inherit some — but not all —

of their parents' genes, they take after their parents in some — but not all — ways. This explains why two very sociable parents can have a child who likes to be alone most of the time, or why two children in the same family can be very different."

"It may be," says Plomin, "that many genes — say ten — contribute to a trait, and having five or six of them is not enough to produce that characteristic. But if you have seven or eight, you're over the brink. That would explain why some children develop their parents' personality problems, and why some children have a problem that neither parent does."

Moreover, other factors must coexist with the predisposing genetic factor for it to be manifested. The knowledge that some personality traits — both positive and negative — as well as some behavior problems have a partial genetic basis is helpful if it relieves parents of the guilt they often feel for not doing everything "right."

"No one is saying that parents are not influential and responsible," Plomin says. "Of course they are. They are just not the *only* influence."

In another study of twins, research conducted at Virginia Commonwealth University under the direction of genetics professor Lindon Eaves examined the differences between behavior, lifestyles, and abilities, as well as why people end up marrying the mates they do. Preliminary findings from the study point to three concepts: personality is hereditary, ideas such as religious beliefs stem from environmental influences, and attitudes on sex and politics are shaped by a combination of both genes and the environment.

"The effect of genes on normal behavior is much more widespread than has been believed." says Eaves. "Most people are not surprised that height runs in the family, but personality does too. The cause is almost all genetic. What our parents give us almost entirely is our genes."

The VCU team has dispelled the popularly held notions that "likes attract" or "opposites attract." "Personality seems to play virtually no role in choosing our mates," says Eaves. Instead, people tend to end up with spouses who share similar socio-economic and educational backgrounds and have similar attitudes on subjects such as politics.

In the Minnesota twins study, the true focus of attention is on genes. What the researchers there hope to discover is the heritability of countless thousands of human traits and characteristics.

"Heritable," they stress, does not mean "*in*heritable." What heritability addresses is percentages — how much, say, our intelligence comes to us in our genes and how much we pick up from our upbringing and our surroundings.

"Just because a characteristic is genetically influenced does not mean it can't be modified," says Nancy Seagal, Minnesota psychologist. "By altering elements of our environment we can alter genetic expression in any number of ways."

This study and others show that a good deal of what we are is inheritable. But heritability figures are estimates, not absolutes. Subsequent experience can sometimes overcome nature.

The Minnesota researchers believe that their findings indicate that mental ability is strongly affected by the genes. However, they do concede that there is no way to separate the development of an inherited trait from its environmental history. They stress, though, that if the environment does influence intellectual abilities, the effect is subtle. Time after time in the Minnesota study, twins with very different schooling opportunities came out only a few points apart in intelligence.

Like intelligence, personality appears to be determined by a complicated interplay of both genes and upbringing. Unlike intelligence, however, temperament traits do not appear to be mainly rooted in the genes. Rather, the formation of personality is closer to a fifty-fifty affair, with genetics and experience both equally important.

Genograms: Patterns for Genealogists

Your family is one of the most powerful influences in your life. To track how feelings and attitudes develop in a family and gauge whether they are causing problems, many family counselors use an exercise called a genogram — a sort of family tree that talks.

A genogram is a format for drawing a family tree that records information about family members and their *relationships* over at least three generations. Genograms display family information graphically.

Genograms originally developed from research on family systems by Murray Bowen, M.D., and are widely used to help people unravel the relationship patterns of their family members and help pinpoint their talents, strengths and weaknesses. They are used by many clinical psychologists dealing with families, but they can be used by everyone as they can help family members see themselves in a new way. A genogram will help you see your family in a "larger picture," both currently and historically. On a genogram, the structural, relational, and functional information about a family can be viewed both horizontally across the family context and vertically through the generations.

One of the fascinations of genograms is how often and how clearly they show relationship patterns recurring across generations. For example, a woman with an alcoholic father may marry a problem drinker herself. She has developed coping skills to deal with a problem that feels familiar to her, and these skills can be transferred easily to a new relationship, even though alcoholism continues to be a disruptive and destructive part of her life.

Genograms encourage you to think about the ways in which the various members of your family get along. Fortunately, you don't need a doctorate to compile a genogram in order to get a broad view of your family. You may not spot and interpret every pattern in your genogram the way a therapist would, but you will see connections you have never seen before. And those insights may prompt you to explore personal difficulties and relationships in a new way.

To create a genogram, go over the key events in your parents' and grandparents' generations — births, marriages, deaths, divorces, household moves, special achievements, financial windfalls or setbacks. What important family events did you witness or hear talked about, and what were the reactions to them? How did your people cope with life transitions — happy turning points as well as difficult times? To draw a basic genogram, you must use the symbols as illustrated in the chart on page 69. First, though, to understand how genograms are used by therapists, study the three genograms of the Adams family.

Diagram A on page 70 shows the successes and failures in the Adams family over four generations, while diagram B on page 70 shows how the expectations of firstborns in this family were passed down, and diagram C on page 71 shows the triangles in John Quincy Adams' life. The joining together of two people in relation to a third defines triangular relationships, and genograms are an extremely handy tool for recognizing them.

Genogram Format And Common Pedigree Symbols

☐   Male

◯   Female

Birth Date ↗79-59↖ ⊠ Death Date   Death=X

▣ ◎   Index Person (IP)

☐m.63◯   Marriage

☐s.72◯   Marital Separation

☐ ◯   Children
☐ ☐ ◯◯   (list in birth order, oldest on left)
65 68 70

◇   Sex Unknown

3   Three Males

⑤   Five Individuals (both sexes)

■   Affected Male

◨   Known Heterozygous Male

⊙   Carrier Female

⬦   Pregnancy In Progress

☐━◯   Consanguineous Marriage

☐━◯   No Known Pregnancy

☐69◯   Living Together Relationship Or Liasion (with date)

☐d.74◯   Divorce (with date)

☐ ◯   Adopted Or Foster Children
◯ ☐

♂◯   Dizygotic (nonidentical) Fraternal Twins

♂◯   Monozygotic (identical) Twins

☐ ◯   Spontaneous Abortion

☐ ◯ ✗   Induced Abortion

☐ ◯ ⊠ ☐   Stillbirth

☐═══◯   Very Close Relationship

☐·····◯   Distant Relationship

☐〰〰◯   Conflictual Relationship

☐┤├◯ 59-64   Estrangement Or Cut Off (give dates if possible)

☐〰〰〰◯   Fused And Conflictual

(Courtesy of Kingdom Productions, Houston, Texas.)

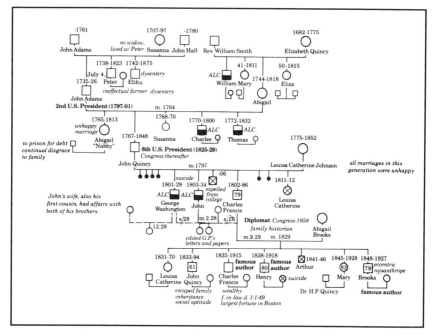

Diagram A. Adams family genogram: successes and failures

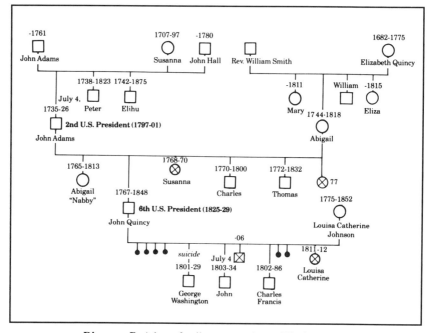

Diagram B. Adams family: expectations of firstborn sons

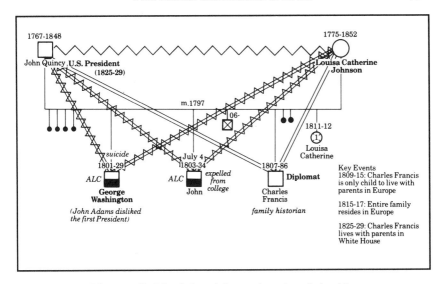

Diagram C. John Quincy Adams: triangular relationships

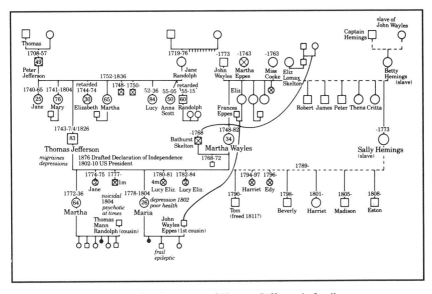

Diagram D. Genogram of Thomas Jefferson's family

Another fascinating genogram is that of Thomas Jefferson, which shows the many interconnected affairs and relationships in his family. (See diagram D on page 71.) This is called a convoluted genogram. Jefferson's daughters, Martha and Maria, both married their cousins. In addition, Martha Jefferson's first husband was the younger brother of her second stepmother's first husband; plus Jefferson's father-in-law had a long relationship with Betty Hemings; and Jefferson had a long relationship and seven children by his slave, Sally Hemings, who was a daughter of Betty.

Now look again at the basic genogram format on page 69. It includes the symbols necessary to describe basic family membership and structure. Your genogram should include the following information about you, your parents and grandparents:

- Name, birthdate and, if deceased, year and cause of death.

- Education and occupation.

- Siblings in each generation. Especially significant is birth order (list oldest to youngest, left to right). Note whether there was a big gap — six years or more — between siblings. Also chart when any deaths, including miscarriages or infant deaths, occurred.

- Marital history, including years of marriages, divorces, deaths of spouses and remarriages. Add anything significant about premarital history (long or broken engagements and long-term and/or live-in relationships, with the year the couple met or started living together if possible).

- Health or psychological problems — chronic illness, heart disease, cancer, alcohol or drug abuse, eating disorders, depression.

Think back to which family members had especially close, distant or difficult relationships and chart these connections as indicated on the keys in the sample genograms. (Remember a relationship can be close *and* difficult at the same time.)

With any genogram data, it's important not to infer too much from isolated facts or characteristics. In addition to looking for cross-generational patterns (such as triangles), check for other potential sources of relationship trouble you might not have considered before. Did any of your family members marry especially late or early? Were the partners at very different life stages? Also check your family history for "coincidences" between events and behavior. Was there a period of prolonged ill health or marital or work stress? How did your people adapt?

Other family information to be noted on a genogram includes:

- ethnic background and migration date
- religion or religious change
- education
- occupation or unemployment
- military service
- retirement
- trouble with the law
- physical abuse or incest
- obesity
- alcohol or drug abuse
- tobacco use
- dates when family members left home
- current location of family members

The genogram also can be used in the management of medical treatment. Family physicians can and sometimes do use their knowledge of patients' family relationships and patterns to develop diagnostic and therapeutic plans. For example, indications of previous illnesses or symptoms patterns on a genogram may lead to early detection of a problem and preventive treatment of family members at risk.

Doing genograms is bound to get you thinking about family life in new ways. We all inherited talents, values, and ways of coping that enabled our parents (and their parents) to endure crises. And though there may be (or may have been) problem relationships in your family, with this method of insight you can change the course of your family history.

5 — Adoption and Your Genetic Roots

Adoption is a subject charged with emotion, and it is difficult to find anyone with an unbiased opinion on whether adoption records should be open, since millions of individuals have been touched by adoption in some way — either as an adoptee, as a birthparent or as an adoptive parent. The number of adoptions in this country in 1985 was estimated at 90,000 and during the 1940s and 1950s the annual numbers reached more than half a million.

The greatest argument for more open records for the millions of adoptees is their basic right to know their genetic roots. For not only do adoptees need to know about their biological backgrounds, but their children and grandchildren want, and need, to know. Past studies indicate that 17 percent of adults who require medical care do so due to genetic problems. For adoptees and their descendants, an accurate family health history is almost impossible to compile, yet they should know about any hereditary diseases and genetic traits their biological parents may have passed on to them.

For anyone considering adoption, priority should be given to obtaining the child's medical history, plus having the door left open so that updated information could be supplied by the biological parent(s), using a third party (the agency, lawyer, etc.) if necessary. Unfortunately, this has not been done in the past. A girl who becomes pregnant at age fifteen probably does not know anything about her own medical history, let alone her family's. However, by the time she is twenty-five or thirty-five she may have acquired information that should be passed on to her adopted child — to warn of disorders or diseases that could affect that child and his or her children. (For this reason, the International Soundex Reunion Register (ISRR) has implemented a medical alert and genetic outreach program in addition to its regular reunion registry. You must be eighteen or older to register. ISRR is located at P.O. Box 2315, Carson City, NV 89702-2312.)

In most cases, for an adoptee to learn about his or her genetic background and family health history, an enormous amount of research not required of others who know their biological origins is necessary. Whether an adoptee decides to locate his or her biological parents, siblings or other relatives is something only the adoptee can decide. But an adoptee can initiate a search to learn about his or her family medical history without having to make a commitment to "find" or seek reunion with biological relatives.

However, an adoptee is faced with the prospect of finding unpleasant things in the process, and a support group is highly recommended before embarking upon a search. In *The Adoption Searchbook*, by Mary Jo Rillera (available from Triadoption Library, P.O. Box 5218, Huntington Beach, CA 92646, or at your local library), the emotions that must be faced and some of the risks are discussed. An adoptee may encounter illness, incest, insanity, incompetence, a different racial background than they were told of, or the fact they may have been the product of rape. Shattered expectations may result.

Another excellent book adoptees and birthparents should read is *Search* by Jayne Askin with Bob Oskam. It will guide you through the complex search process.

Two inexpensive packages of booklets, prepared by Concerned United Birthparents (CUB), are available through People Searching News, P.O. Box 22611, Fort Lauderdale, FL 33335-2611. One is the Adoptee package and the other is the Birthparent package. These booklets deal with such topics as: "Thoughts for Birthparents Newly Considering Search," "The Post-adoption Experience of Surrendering Parents," "Birthparents Searching: You Can't Have it Both Ways," and "Thoughts to Consider for Newly Searching Adoptees."

Two other references, especially slanted for the adoptee's research problems, are: *The New ISC Searchbook* and *Faint Trails*. These are available also through People Searching News, which publishes a reference magazine for adoption, genealogical searches and missing person searches six times per year.

Sources of Information

For the adoptee who wishes to learn primarily about his or her family medical history, the place to start is with the adoptive parents. They will have some knowledge of the surrender or adoption and the people, places and dates involved. In addition, there are usually other family members who have a few memories that can provide clues to unlocking the puzzle. These memories should be compiled in a written form so they can be used as reference. Interview relatives and other individuals who may have been part of any phase of the placement. You need all the clues you can get.

Nearly all states have a central adoption unit where files are kept on all surrenders and adoptions initiated or concluded there. Each state files a variety of information. The records are slightly different from year to year and state to state and even depend on the persons who filed the data, but they probably will include the following:

- Original certificate of birth
- Amended certificate of birth
- Relinquishment, consent and surrender papers
- Petition to adopt
- Case or home study information
- Final adoption decree

All states have a centralized vital records office in the capital city. However, county and city bureaus still exist and often have older or duplicate records. In the majority of states the original certificate of birth is considered "sealed" after an adoption is finalized and will not be released without a court order. Many laws pertaining to vital records have been passed in recent years and do not have a retroactive effect. It may be necessary to check the state statutes and the years they became law.

In vital records offices you will find the following:

- Original certificate of birth
- Amended certificate of birth
- Death certificate
- Marriage license and application
- Some divorce records

There are public and private placement agencies that may have been involved in any or all phases of adoption. They must be licensed by the state. Even in a so-called "independent" adoption (where the child is surrendered to the adoptive parents directly) a state or county worker is usually assigned by the court to review the prospective adoptive home before the finalization. Agency files vary in detail and format. Old files may have been transferred to microfilm. These files may include the following:

- Background information on birth family
- Medical information on birth family
- Original certificate of birth
- Amended certificate of birth
- Medical or foster care consent
- Relinquishment, surrender or termination of parental rights
- Psychological testing of birthparents
- Psychological testing of child
- Medical records of birthmother and child
- Petition to adopt
- Interlocutory (if issued)
- Home study of prospective parents
- Foster care information
- Adoption decree
- Adoption certificate
- Follow-up or future contacts and updates made by any parties involved

The court having jurisdiction in an adoption is the court in the county where the adopting parents reside, where the adoptee resided, or where the placing agency was located. This court continues to have authority over matters pertaining to the adoption. The court files usually contain the following documents and reports:

- Petition to adopt
- Interlocutory (if issued)
- Original certificate of birth
- Surrender, relinquishment or termination of parental rights
- Home study report by social worker
- Final adoption decree
- Adoption certificate (if issued)

If a maternity home is involved there will be records pertaining primarily to the birthmother. Occasionally there will be limited information on the child if born in residence and kept for a few days or weeks. Often these records are destroyed after a few years, or when the home closes, but sometimes they are transferred to another agency, church or hospital. If a birthmother used a false identity in all other records, these files may reveal her true name.

The hospital where the child was born will have medical and delivery records. Often they are stored in some remote place or transferred to microfilm. Even if the files were destroyed (which happens rarely) there will be separate admittance records which could supply names and addresses. Medical and delivery files contain a variety of information such as addresses, next- of-kin, financial payments, pre- and post-natal care, footprints, medical history and sometimes the original birth certificate.

Doctors who gave pre- and post-natal care and the doctor at delivery will often keep their own records. These are separate from the hospital records unless they did not have a private practice. These too will supply names, addresses, next-of-kin, payments, medical care and history. In an independent adoption where the doctor was instrumental in placement, the files often contain information on the adoptive parents as well.

In nearly all adoptions there will be an attorney representing the petitioners. In a private or independent adoption the lawyer or law firm will be serving both the birthparents and adoptive parents. In either case, there will be a file containing most of the following:

- Petition to adopt
- Interlocutory (if issued)
- Adoption decree
- Surrender, relinquishment or termination of parental rights
- Original certificate of birth
- Amended certificate of birth
- Financial arrangements

The documents and records that an adoptee needs most to learn about his or her family medical history are the very ones that are most difficult to obtain. For example, the original birth certificate, which is issued shortly after delivery and prior to adoption being finalized, often contains valuable information on the birth family. This information may include the birthmother's maiden name, the birthfather's name, their occupations, previous births to this mother and the name of the doctor or other person attending the birth.

When an adoption is finalized, the original birth certificate is closed or "sealed" and an amended certificate is issued in its place. State laws vary on the availability of the original certificate. The original birth record may be held by city, county or state vital records offices as well as the agency, the state department concerned, and the court. Finding and obtaining this document is one of the most difficult aspects of genealogical research for an adoptee. You may need professional help to aid you in this.

Surrender, relinquishment or consent to adopt papers are documents which were signed by the birthparent(s) severing their parental rights and responsibilities. Termination of parental rights can also be done by a court order when the birthparent(s) are not willing to surrender custody of their child, or the court has seen evidence of abuse, neglect or abandonment. You will find these documents, or copies of them, in the court, agency or state department files. Also the lawyer for the petitioners or the lawyer in an independent adoption usually will have copies of these documents in their files.

The surrender or relinquishment documents will give the birthparent(s)' name(s), possibly the child's birth name, the agency involved, and usually an address of the birthparent(s). The consent to adopt will usually give birthparent(s)' name(s), adoptive parent(s)' name(s) and the child's name. Termination of parental rights will state the reason for termination, birthparent(s)' name(s), some addresses or places of usual residence and ages — all clues which the adoptee can use to conduct further research.

An adoption decree is kept in the court files in the court that had jurisdiction in the adoption. Though many agencies, state departments and lawyers have copies, they are often reluctant to release them. This decree will state the adoptive parent(s)' name(s), the child's adoptive name, and usually the birthparent(s)' name(s) and the birth name of the child. In most states these decrees are available only to the parties to the action. This means that the birthparent(s), adoptive parent(s) and the adoptee could, in most cases, obtain a copy from the clerk of the court.

The adopting parents must file a petition to adopt with the local court. The court may issue an interlocutory until the waiting period has passed (in most states from six months to one year). At that time the court reviews the petition and issues a final decree of adoption.

Finding hospital records is not easy, but you should check the amended birth certificate first. Usually the physician will be listed and the hospital he or she worked at can be established by calling the area hospitals or the area medical association. The hospital will be listed on the original birth certificate. Or you can ask the agency, state department or lawyer(s) involved in the adoption. If all else fails do a blanket search of all hospitals in the area. Some hospitals will not release their medical files to an individual but will release them to a physician. You may need to enlist the aid of your own physician. If there is a possibility of genetic disease, your physician will probably aid you in your search.

Maternity hospitals are the least cooperative in releasing files. Often the files are in storage and frequently the clerks will tell you that the records have been destroyed. However, *seldom* do hospitals actually destroy their records. If the medical records have been destroyed, there will still be an admittance record, and it should show the name(s) of the birthparent(s), residence, age and date of admittance, and of course the financial arrangements. Many hospitals also issue an admittance record on the infant shortly after birth. You may also discover on the admittance records such information as birth grandparent(s)' names, ages, occupations, places and dates of birth, education, religion and residence, as well as information about the adoptive parents.

Hospital records may have information about the birthmother — her name, address, date admitted, time admitted, age, place and date of birth, husband or other responsible party, employer, occupation, nest-of-kin or friend, doctor who delivered, financial arrangements, insurance company and medical diagnosis, treatment and discharge. When requesting hospital records, it is best not to mention adoption.

State Records

Most states have a central adoption unit that keeps very thorough information on each surrender and adoption that takes place within their state. If there was an agency involved, this department would be able to identify the agency and the current address. If the agency is no longer in existence, this department will be able to tell a searcher where the records are now held. If a private or independent adoption is involved, the state unit will have the records and can tell the searcher how to get the information they want.

State records may include the following: birthparent(s)' names, ages, residences, places and dates of birth; birth grandparents' names, ages and usual state of residency; birth medical history; hospital of birth; foster care; adoptive parent(s)' names, ages, residence, occupations, places and dates of birth, educational background and medical history; court of jurisdiction, and agency or lawyer involved.

Other documents that are normally included in state files are the original and amended birth certificates, the surrender, relinquishment or consent to adopt, the petition to adopt and the adoption decree. However, the state may ask that you contact the agency or the court to get copies of them.

Most adoptees do not have a copy of their original birth certificate, which gives the name(s) of their birthparent(s). This document is critical to research for genealogical and medical purposes, since you cannot find your biological families without names. Some states will release the original birth certificate to adult adoptees upon request. Other states will not. Some will deny it exists or will require a court order for its release. Contact (write or visit) the bureau of vital records in your city, county and state of birth. Each bureau will respond differently and one may give you the certificate you want. However, in order to request an original birth certificate, you must know what your surname was at birth.

Check at your local library for the following booklet (also available, for a nominal fee, from the Superintendent of Documents, U.S. Government Printing Office, Washington, DC 20402): "Where to Write for Vital Records" (birth, death, marriage and divorce).

Another handy reference is *Vital Records Handbook*, by Thomas J. Kemp, published in 1988 by the Genealogical Publishing Company of Baltimore. It not only lists the names of the vital statistics departments in each state, but tells you the dates for which birth, marriage and death records are available and the costs of these documents. Of course, prices are always subject to change, but this book will also give you a copy of the forms each of these bureaus uses. Simply photocopy the form, fill it out and send the stated fee to the proper bureau. If the prices have changed, you will be notified and you can remit the additional amount.

In addition to listing each state, the *Vital Records Handbook* has information for American Samoa, Guam, the Panama Canal Zone, Puerto Rico, the Virgin Islands — St. Croix, St. Thomas and St. John — Canada (all provinces), Ireland, England and Wales, Northern Ireland, and Scotland.

The adoption decree is available to adoptees in nearly every state. Check first with your family or the family lawyer to see if there is a copy of this document. If these sources fail you, then write to the county clerk and for a small fee you should be able to get a copy. If there is any altering or marking out of important information done on this document, you may want to contact an adoptee movement group for assistance.

You should also ask for the petition to adopt along with the adoption decree. These are two different documents, but should be acquired.

Surrender, relinquishment, consent to adopt and termination of parental rights are difficult documents to obtain. Possibly the adoptive parents or their attorney have copies and will be willing to share with you. Most agencies, states and courts will refuse to release these documents to the adoptee because they reveal the birthparent(s)' name(s). However, some judges will see that they are included in the court-ordered released files.

Other Records

Hospital records are not always easy to obtain either. If you have your birthmother's name at the time of your birth, you may be able to get the hospital records. It is possible that you can get these records with just the birthdate and your present name. Some adoptees have found that a personal visit or a phone call will expedite matters. You may be told that these records will only be released to your physician. In that case, enlist the aid of your family doctor and ask him or her to let you see the records when they arrive. If your physician is not helpful you can research the state law concerning release of medical records to see if you can force their release to you, or contact a movement group who may know a doctor who will help you.

If yours was an independent adoption, or if you do not know the agency, the court or the present location of your files, write to the state department in the state in which you were born and/or adopted. If your state does not keep centralized files on adoptions they will inform you. Then you may have to resort to letter writing to determine the agency, court, hospital, etc.

If your adoption was handled by an agency, there is usually an abundance of information available from them. You may be able to ascertain a great deal of medical, genetic and personal history information from their files.

Some courts are willing to respond to all adoptee requests for the opening of the sealed records, while other courts do it only in the event of extreme medical necessity or in matters relating to inheritance. Adoption groups usually know about the responsiveness of the courts in their areas. It never hurts to try. You do not need a lawyer. Some courts have a form to fill out, and if you write to them they will send you a copy of this form. The request for medical information about one's biological parents is good cause to have court records opened for you, and you just may be able to get the information you need by writing to the court. Some judges are quite sympathetic to adoptees, especially when medical problems threaten them or their children.

Birthparents

If you are a birthparent, you may need to contact the court in order to supply your adopted child with medical information. Otherwise you should contact the agency or state department involved and supply any medical or genetic background material which you have learned about yourself and your child's biological ancestors. Request that this information be given to the adoptee, and hopefully the adoptee will be contacted or will try to obtain this information on his own.

If you ever used an alias or a false identity during your association with the adoption agency, maternity home, hospital, doctor, lawyer or any other information source, correct that information. If you gave any type of inaccurate or false information about the birthfather or mother, correct that too. It is difficult to amend or correct information without seeing what is already held in the files, so if you can get or view complete copies it will help you give accurate or updated information.

Genealogical Research Tips for Adoptees

When a petition to adopt is filed in any court, proper notice must be given to the birthparents or legal guardians of the child. However, when birthparents surrender the child to an agency or consent to the adoption by a specific couple, they often waive their right to notification. In the past, the alleged father did not have to be notified. However, since 1972 birthfathers have had more rights, and in most states notification is now required. If the court or its representatives are not able to notify the birthparent directly, they must publish a notice of the intent to adopt in a newspaper in the area where the parent is known to have last resided.

If you know in which county the adoption was filed, and if you know the approximate date the petition was filed, you can search through the newspapers that carried legal notices in that county. If birth and adoption counties are different, search in both counties. If a notice was required, it should have been published from a month or two after the petition to adopt was filed up to the month just prior to the final order of adoption.

The great value of these legal notices is that they may provide you with the legal name not only of your birthmother, but also of your birthfather.

The newspapers will not research this information for you. However, by writing to the city or county library where the adoption was filed or the birth occurred, you can learn if these newspapers are on file (usually in microform). Also many libraries keep a vertical file relating to birth, death and marriage records in their locality. You can also write to the genealogical society in that county and ask for the name of a researcher who would be willing to undertake this search of legal notices for you. Or if the newspapers you need have been microfilmed (usually the state library or archives will have them), you may be able to borrow copies through interlibrary loan and read them for yourself.

You may be able to learn more about your birthparent(s) by utilizing school and alumni records. If you know the approximate years of attendance in some high school or college, you may be able to get information from school and alumni records or the yearbooks. School records will often be released to a family member doing genealogical research. Just state your relationship and ask for the specific information you want. However, don't mention adoption. School policies can differ greatly and you may have to try several different approaches.

School reunion committees may be able to help you and you may be able to find pictures of your birthparents simply by locating copies of old yearbooks and doing a bit of sleuthing.

City directories can be especially useful in tracking your birthparents (and your grandparents). From them you will get an idea of the family, where they lived, when they moved, married, died, and their occupations. Most county or city libraries keep back issues of directories for their areas, and the LDS (Mormon) Family History Library in Salt Lake City has many old city directories on microfilm.

When researching in city directories make sure to check the symbol pages in the front section. There are different symbols and abbreviations which you must know in order to get the most from the directory. The listings of businesses, institutions and professions that many contain can be useful when you need to do a blanket mailing to hospitals, churches, doctors, schools, and so on. Most libraries will answer your request by mail for information from their city directories. Send a few dollars to pay for the photocopying fees and a self-addressed, stamped No. 10 envelope.

Another source which an adoptee may have recourse to in locating a birthparent or grandparent is the Social Security Administration. SSA will forward non-threatening letters for you. Write your brief letter, put it in an *unsealed* stamped envelope with the person's name on the envelope; then write a letter to SSA, put all of this in another envelope and send it to: Location Services, Social Security Administration, 6401 Security Blvd., Baltimore, MD 21235. In your letter to SSA say: Please forward the enclosed letter to (name of person), whose last known address was (full-address, if known; or city and state). If it is a common name, you may need to include additional information (like birthdate) to help SSA identify the person.

Insurance Records

If you come across the name of an insurance company while searching for medical and/or adoption records, you should follow up on it. Insurance records are of great value. Companies have various methods of keeping records and the type of insurance policy will dictate what data is compiled on an individual. However, all insurance records will have Social Security numbers, date and place of birth, address and full names. Life and health insurance will have additional data such as beneficiaries named, conversions made, payments, if any, and to whom they were made. Health and dental plans will have records of payment for illness and medical care, type of problem and where treated, next-of-kin, place of employment and previous health problems.

Insurance companies all have different policies regarding requests for information. When dealing with them, remember to emphasize that the person you are inquiring about is a close relative, and don't mention adoption.

Adoptees may need to check a U.S. census record that is later than 1910 (the most recent census open to researchers). To obtain information that is less than seventy-five years old from the Bureau of the Census, the searcher must have the full birth name, and the purpose must be to prove the age and identity of someone. Two census searches can be done for one fee. In the letter of inquiry, you should add to the information anything you feel will help the census bureau positively identify the person. Information on brothers, sisters, parents' death, divorce, separation, step-parents and alternate addresses may be helpful. Write to: United States Department of Commerce, Bureau of the Census, Pittsburg, KS 66762 for forms, fees and complete instructions.

Death Records and Obituaries

Death records may supply you with important medical information and information about the deceased's parents — all significant genealogical data. Most death certificates are filed at the state level, though some are available from the county. Check the *Vital Records Handbook* for information and forms.

You should search for obituaries about your family members — all of them, not just your direct line — for many of the earlier obituaries contain a great deal of information about the person, sometimes even the diseases that afflicted him. Obituaries are also rich sources for learning the names and places of residence of family members, parents' names, dates of birth and death, religious affiliation, where buried and the funeral home involved. All this can lead to a great deal more genealogical information.

The funeral home should have the name of any insurance company that made payment for services rendered and the name of any insurance company with which the deceased held a policy. While these are not public records, funeral homes will usually share this information with you.

Checklist

A checklist for adoptees to help locate information about their birthparents includes:

Adoption Papers

> —Change of Name
> —Finalized Court Papers
> —Home Study Report
> —Petition to Adopt
> —Relinquishment Papers

Agency Records

> —Application to Adopt
> —Baptism Certificate
> —Financial Agreements
> —Foster Homes
> —Home Study Report
> —Medical Information
> —Petition to Adopt
> —Relinquishment Papers

Birth Records

> —Altered Certificate
> —Baptism or Christening Certificate
> —Original Certificate
> —Published Birth Notice

Court Records

> —Adoption Records
> —Change of Name
> —Citizenship
> —Relinquishment Records

Family Records

—Correspondence

—Insurance Records

—Photographs

—Bibles, Baby Books

Hospital Records

—Admittance

—Delivery Room

—Medical Records

—Nursery Records

—Release Records

Newspapers

—Engagements

—Graduations

—Military Service Notes

—Obituaries

—Published Births

—Published Deaths

—Published Divorces

—Published Marriages

—Notification of Birthparent(s)

The following organizations can be contacted for additional information:

People Searching News, P.O. Box 22611, Fort Lauderdale, FL 33335-2611.

The ALMA Society, P.O. Box 154, Washington Bridge Station, New York, NY 10033.

American Adoption Congress, P.O. Box 44040, L'Enfant Plaza Station, Washington, DC 20026.

Concerned United Birthparents, 2000 Walker St., Des Moines, IA 50317.

International Soundex Reunion Register, P.O.Box 2312, Carson City, NV 89702-2312.

6 — Tips for Researching Your Medical Pedigree

I t is not necessary that you become a genealogist to compile a medical pedigree, for actually you need only concern yourself with gaining accurate medical information about your families as far back as your four grandparents. But you will need to do this on your side of the family as well as your spouse's in order to provide your children with a family health tree. If you can trace lines to the eight great-grandparents on each side, so much the better. The major records you need to locate, analyze and compile for your family health tree include:

- Death certificates
- Newspaper obituaries
- Insurance company records
- Hospital records
- Medical records
- Census records
- Mortality schedules
- Military records

Death Certificates

Death certificates are modern records and most of them are available from state offices, called vital statistics offices, which are usually part of each state's Department of Health and Social Services. The titles of these offices vary from state to state, but for the most part a Bureau of Vital Statistics located in the capital city will have these records.

Costs for certified copies of death certificates range from about $5 to as much $20, and obtaining one for each of your grandparents and parents can be a considerable expense. You should check first to see if any copies of death certificates exist among family members. This can save you money and eliminate obtaining duplicate copies. All you want to know is what your ancestors died of and any contributing disease that may appear on the records. For this purpose it is not necessary to have a certified copy, so in some instances you need only request a duplicate copy of a death certificate; these are usually much cheaper than a certified copy.

The dates that death certificates are available for will also vary from state to state. Some states, like Delaware, have death records that date from as early as 1861, but most state records begin in the early 1900s. First you need to determine the approximate date your ancestor died and the state in which he or she died — not the state where he or she is buried necessarily. Then you can consult a pamphlet, available in most libraries, entitled "Where to Write for Vital Records", published by the U.S. Department of Health and Human Services. Another excellent source for this information is Thomas J. Kemp's *Vital Records Handbook* (1988), described in the previous chapter. It gives you the name of each state repository that has the records, its address, the price of these documents (as of the publication date), plus forms you can use to request the death certificates.

If your ancestor was a U.S. citizen and died in a foreign country, the death would normally have been reported to the nearest U.S. consular office. The consul prepared an official "Report of the Death of an American Citizen Abroad" and a copy of the report of death was filed permanently in the U.S. Department of State. To obtain a copy of a report, write to Passport Services, Correspondence Branch, U.S. Department of State, Washington, DC 20523. The fee for a copy is about $4. However, if your ancestor was a member of the armed forces of the United States, attached at the time of death to the Army, Navy, Air Force or Coast Guard, the records will be elsewhere. For members of the Army, Navy or Air Force, write to the Secretary of Defense, Washington, DC

20301. For members of the Coast Guard, write to the Commandant, P.S., U.S. Coast Guard, Washington, DC 20226.

When a death occurs on the high seas, whether in an aircraft or on a vessel, the determination of where the record is filed is decided by the direction in which the vessel or aircraft was headed at the time of the event. If the vessel or aircraft was outbound or docked or landed at a foreign port, requests for copies of the records should be made to the U.S. Department of State, Washington, DC 20520. If the vessel or aircraft was inbound and the first port of entry was in the United States, write to the registration authority in the city where the vessel or aircraft docked or landed in the United States. If the vessel was of U.S. registry, contact the U.S. Coast Guard facility at the port of entry.

Most, but not all, foreign countries record births and deaths, and most will provide certificates of births and deaths occurring within their boundaries. U.S. citizens who need a copy of a foreign death record may obtain assistance by writing to the Office of Overseas Citizens Services, U.S. Department of State, Washington, DC 20520. Aliens residing in the United States who seek records of these events should contact their nearest consular office.

The U.S. Department of Health, Education and Welfare, Public Health Service, also has the booklet — mentioned above — "Where to Write for Vital Records." It includes information on where to write for birth and death records of U.S. citizens who were born or died outside the United States and where to write for birth certificates for alien children adopted by U.S. citizens. It is available from the Superintendent of Documents, U.S. Government Printing Office, Washington, DC 20402.

Death certificates for all parents, grandparents and their siblings should be obtained in order to compile an accurate family health tree. Your grandfather may have died accidentally or from a disease that is non-genetic. However, all or some of his brothers and sisters may have suffered from diabetes or heart attacks, and it is important to have this information.

If your ancestors died in a large city in the United States, you may discover death records are available much earlier than the state records. For example, Baltimore has them dating from 1875 and New Orleans from 1803. New York City's boroughs vary. They include the Bronx from 1899 (with records from 1866 to 1897 in Manhattan), Brooklyn (deaths in Kings County from 1847, others in the City Health Department from 1866), and Manhattan from 1866 (deaths from 1847) at the Municipal Archives, New York Public Library. Philadelphia from 1860, Pittsburgh from 1870, and Albany, Buffalo and Yonkers, New York have records earlier than the state records, which date from 1914.

There also are a few states which have early vital records that are collected and indexed in their state libraries and archives, and some of them are published. If you need death records of ancestors who died in the following areas, for example, check these additional sources:

- **Connecticut** — The Barbour Collection of vital records compiled from church, cemetery and town records prior to 1850.

- **Delaware** — Death records from 1855 to 1910 (with a card index to records from very early to 1888) are at the Hall of Records in Dover.

- **Maine** — Records for eighty towns, with vital records index. Check with the Maine Historical Society in Portland.

- **Maryland** — Deaths from 1865 to 1880; indexes are in the Hall of Records in Annapolis.

- **Massachusetts** — From early to 1850, church and cemetery records for more than 200 towns have been published, mostly by the New England Historic Genealogical Society and the Essex Institute.

- **New Hampshire** — Town records from the 1850s, indexed in a special collection at the State House in Concord.

- **Rhode Island** — The Arnold Collection of Vital Records (1636 to 1850) is published in twenty-one volumes, and is available in many libraries.

- **Vermont** — An index to vital records from early to 1870 and also one from 1871 to 1908 can be found at the Secretary of State's Office, Montpelier.

There are some problems with death certificates and records. Generally they were completed with information provided by a particular informant, usually a family member, and the information may be accurate and it may not be. However, while the other genealogical data may not be completely accurate, the data pertaining to the cause of death was normally provided by the attending physician and will be accurate, and that is the information you are seeking to compile a family health tree.

Information on death certificates will not only include the date and cause of death but also provide you with the age at which your ancestor died and the name of the funeral home, if applicable. The cause of death may be pulmonary edema, and any condition which gave rise to immediate cause is often noted, such as "senility", or it may say cause of death was "angina pectoris" with influenza as a contributory cause. The length of illness also is usually noted.

Once you have obtained death certificates or information about your ancestors' health from other records, you can compile this information listing your ancestors' names, dates of death, ages and causes of death. The compilation of this information often reveals patterns. That is, you may discover that on your father's side most of your ancestors died of heart-related diseases and that on your mother's side cancer was prevalent. Or you may discover that most of your family died simply of "old age" or accidental causes.

Newspaper Obituaries and Other Records

Other records to find and use that may contain information about the causes of your ancestor' deaths are: newspaper obituaries, funeral notices, cemetery records, tombstones, mortuary records, masonic records, family Bibles, and old letters. Churches sometimes kept funeral records and it may also be necessary to check coroners' records or inquests. Hospitals and doctors keep all sorts of health records.

Some cemetery records contain information as to the cause of death. These records can be found in the sexton's office, and you should ask to see them — just in case there is additional data about your ancestors. Some cemeteries kept rather detailed records of the diseases and debilities of our ancestors, at least for a certain time period, and if such information exists, you'll want to obtain it.

Obituaries, especially in older newspapers, often identify the diseases from which our ancestors suffered. In more recent obituaries you may not find this information, but an important clue may lie in the type of organization the family suggested memorial contributions be made to — Heart Fund, Cancer Fund, etc. While not reliable as to the cause of death, these notations may be an indication that your ancestor died or suffered from heart disease or cancer, for example.

Insurance Company Records

Life insurance records can be interesting for genealogists and may provide significant information pertaining to the health, age and lifestyle of your ancestors. As early as 1865 medical information on diseases or health condition was included on insurance policies. In 1889, Mutual Life began attaching a medical examination to its policy. Since life insurance is usually paid after the death of the insured, the companies kept their records for many years. To protect themselves legally, most companies kept their records long past the death of the insured. However, these are private records, and for the genealogist they can be most difficult to find and obtain access to. Most older insurance companies still exist — perhaps under a new name — but they usually will not search their large files for you.

Most of these records are in corporation archives, and if you write to the home office they may aid you in locating the material. Be prepared to do the research yourself, however, and to show proof of descent from the relevant ancestor. Also a current agent of the company may help you gain access to old records, especially if you tell him or her about your interest in compiling a family health tree.

The best way to learn which company insured your ancestor is by checking with living family members. They may have old insurance certificates or other information among family papers that will give you the information you need.

For a list of life insurance companies commencing business prior to 1876 and in active operation in 1942 consult *The Source: A Guidebook of American Genealogy*, ed. Arlene Eakle and Johni Cerny (Salt Lake City: Ancestry Pub., 1984). It will give you the names, home office and date of founding for each one of the companies listed.

Hospital and Medical Records

These are among the most difficult to locate and access. Often they will not be made available even to immediate family members. However, your personal physician can probably obtain copies of them — especially if you discover there are genetic disorders in your family. Enlist his or her aid to get this information.

Normally, hospital registers will tell you the patient's name, age, birthplace, date of admission, illness or disease, and date of discharge or death.

The names of general hospitals and their addresses and phone numbers in the United States can be obtained by consulting the *National Yellow Book*, a directory available in most public libraries. It also lists Veteran Administration (VA) hospitals and the names of funeral directors.

Death certificates will give the name and address of the hospital where a person died (providing the person was in a hospital at the time of death). Using this information, you can then try to obtain the admittance record, which usually contains vital data such as Social Security number, insurance information and policy numbers, names of relatives and conventional biographical data. A patient's history will often reveal the number of his or her siblings and the ages the parents were at their death.

Send your request to the Medical Records Department of the hospital along with proof of death (a photocopy of the death certificate or even a tombstone photograph) and ask for a copy of the admittance record and patient history. However, a word of caution. Do not order an *entire* medical record without first getting an estimate of costs. It could be lengthy and expensive. And if the hospital will not release the records to you, enlist the aid of your family doctor.

Census Records

While census records exist in the United States dating back to 1790, for the purpose of obtaining information about your family's health the ones you will be most concerned with are fairly recent — dating back from 1910 (the most recent available to the public at this date) to 1850.

Census records are among those records most commonly used by genealogists and they will provide you with a great deal of information about your ancestors. But for now, the main consideration is the health and medical data available in them.

The 1910 and 1900 censuses are most valuable. Begin your research with them. These records are available in the National Archives in Washington, DC and in all eleven of its regional branches located in the metropolitan areas of Atlanta, Boston, Chicago, Denver, Fort Worth, Kansas City, Los Angeles, New York City, Philadelphia, San Francisco, and Seattle. They can also be obtained through the LDS Family History Library in Salt Lake City, Utah, and its hundreds of branch libraries throughout the country, and through many public libraries.

1910 Census — The 1910 Federal Population Census asked a number of questions that will provide vital information about your families. However, the questions relating to health were minimal. It asked if a person was blind in both eyes or deaf and dumb. Answers to these questions pertaining to family members may give you clues to possible genetic diseases that exist in your family. Of course blindness and deafness could have been the result of accidents or other diseases and not genetic in origin. Use such answers only as a guide.

Some genealogists have traced hereditary deafness in the family by searching through the census records and noting the number of occurrences of deafness and then used other modern records to establish that the deafness was probably genetic. If you discover a number of your ancestors were listed as blind after they reached middle-age, possibly the cause was glaucoma, which could alert you to the likelihood that the disease may "run in the family."

1900 Census — While the 1900 census is one of the most valuable for genealogists because it answers many basic genealogical questions, it does not contain much information useful for a family health tree other than how many children your female ancestor gave birth to and how many were living in 1900. That information could alert you to the possibility of "female problems" if you discover the ancestress gave birth to eight children but only one or two survived. While not documented proof that there was a reproduction problem, since many families lost children to childhood diseases that have since been eradicated, any clue to such problems should be noted and researched by using other records.

1890 Census — This census was 99-percent destroyed in a fire in 1921 and only portions of it exist. This was an unfortunate loss since this census asked about chronic or acute diseases and whether an individual was crippled, maimed or deformed (with name of defect). The surviving fragments have been indexed and both census and index microfilmed, and they are available at all branches of the National Archives. You might be fortunate and find some of your families on it.

One important supplemental schedule for this time period does exist. It is called the Special Schedule of Pensioners, 1890. This special schedule of inquiry lists the names, organizations, and length of service of those who had served in the Army, Navy, or Marine Corps in the Civil War and who were alive at the time of said inquiry, or whose widows were alive. Among the items called for was information about disability, if any.

Unfortunately, practically all of the schedules for the states (alphabetically) from Alabama through Kansas, and about one-half of Kentucky, were apparently destroyed. The extant records can be found at the National Archives and its branches under Special Schedules of the Eleventh Census (1890) Enumerating Union Veterans and Widows of Union Veterans of the Civil War. Occasionally, Confederate veterans were enumerated in the Southern states, and you will find their names and entries, even though crossed out by census checkers, quite legible.

1880 Census — This census enables you to begin tracing some genetic symptoms and diseases. It asked about illness or disability on the day of the census and is the first census to state everyone's relationship to the head of household. It also asked whether persons were deaf, dumb, blind or insane.

1870 Census — This asked whether a person was deaf, dumb, blind or insane and whether a person was a survivor of the Civil War, which can lead you to the military and pension records that may contain family health data, and also alert you to check for your ancestor and/or his widow in the special 1890 schedule mentioned above.

1850 and 1860 Censuses — Both of these censuses have columns relating to whether a person was deaf, dumb, blind or insane

Many genealogists, especially early in their research, neglect to record certain portions of a census. If you failed to note all the information, particularly the medically relevant material, you should go back and re-check censuses to be sure you have recorded all the data found in each census.

Special Federal Schedules — Under an Act of March 3, 1879, which provided that any state could take an interdecennial census with partial reimbursement by the federal government, Colorado, Florida, Nebraska and the territories of Dakota and New Mexico (which included Arizona at that time) did so and returned these schedules to the Secretary of the Interior. Schedule No. 1 identified each inhabitant, occupation and kind of sickness or disability, if any. Schedule No. 5 was a mortality schedule which gave the cause of death for every person who died within the year ending May 31, 1885.

These schedules are interfiled and arranged alphabetically by state and then by county. Many counties are missing. The National Archives holds the originals and has microfilmed the ones for Colorado and Nebraska.

Mortality Schedules, 1850-85

Mortality schedules were conceived for the purpose of collecting information about births, marriages and deaths. They should not be overlooked. They are not complete — probably only 60 percent of the actual deaths were reported — but they can be extremely useful in compiling data about the cause of death of some of your ancestors. While you may not find your direct line in any of these records, you should extract the names of all possible family members. If you have done your genealogical homework, you may recognize the names of the men your ancestor's sisters married.

In 1918 and 1919 these mortality schedules, with the exception of those for 1885, were removed from federal custody and each state was given the option of securing the ones relating to it. Those not claimed by the states were given to the National Society of the Daughters of the American Revolution (DAR) and were placed in its library in Washington, DC. The original schedules held by the DAR are for the states of Arizona, Colorado, Georgia, Kentucky, Louisiana, Tennessee and the District of Columbia. Most have been indexed by the DAR and some have been transcribed. All of the 1885 schedules are in the National Archives except those for Dakota, which are in the library of the North Dakota State Historical Society at Bismarck.

The federal mortality schedules for Arizona, Colorado, District of Columbia, Georgia, Kentucky, Louisiana and Tennessee have been reproduced as microfilm publication T655, *Federal Mortality Census Schedules, 1850-80, and Related Indexes in the Custody of the Daughters of the American Revolution.* This microfilm publication is found at the Chicago, Denver and Los Angeles branches of the National Archives. Other branch holdings of mortality schedules on microfilm or in printed form include Iowa (1850-80), Nebraska (1860 and 1870) and Kansas (1860-80) at the Kansas City Branch; and Virginia (1850-80) at the Philadelphia Branch.

Consult the *Guide to Genealogical Research in the National Archives* (Washington, DC: National Archives, 1982) for a list of mortality schedules by state available through the National Archives and its regional branches.

Most of the mortality schedules are also available through the LDS Family History Library and its branches and will be found on microfiche. To determine the ones available check the Family History Library Catalog at any branch library under [State]/Census or [State]/Vital Records.

Mortality schedules cover dates for the year prior to the federal census. That is, the 1850 mortality schedules supposedly cover deaths from 1 June 1849 through May of 1850. However, there are exceptions to these dates, so you should check the schedules if any of your family died any time during the 1849 to 1850 time period. The information in them includes the name of the person, his or her age, sex, state of birth, month of death, cause of death, profession/occupation/trade, and number of days ill. In the 1880 mortality schedule the place where the disease was contracted was added.

Mortality schedules are useful for tracing and documenting genetic symptoms and diseases. By using these schedules to document death dates of family members, you can follow up with focused searches in obituaries, mortuary records, and cemeteries.

Military Records

Military records pertaining to your ancestors may provide some information about the diseases your ancestors suffered from.

To obtain copies of veterans' records use NATF Form 80, available from the National Archives, to request a search of the records. Complete the form and mail to: Military Service Branch (NNMS), National Archives and Records Service, 8th and Pennsylvania Avenue, N.W., Washington, DC 20408.

Service records and pension records for those who served in World War I and later wars are not available for public searching, though some information can be obtained under certain conditions. Using records for soldiers who served within the past seventy-five years is restricted to immediate family under the provisions of the Right-to-Privacy Acts. Most of the federal records in this category are housed at the National Personnel Records Center, 9700 Page Boulevard, St. Louis, MO 63123. Living veterans can request their records or give written consent to others.

For complete information on the enormous amount of material available about veterans read the chapter on military records in *The Source.*

Using Your Sources

The foregoing are the main records available to you to enable you to compile an accurate family health tree. However, the number one thing to do is to talk to family members about medical problems that your family has had. Pay attention to family traditions about health problems. Take careful notes and then take this information to your family physician. He or she can help you translate medical terms and analyze the information as it applies to you and your descendants.

The major diseases you should be concerned with, since they affect 80 percent of the population, are heart disease, cancer and diabetes. Using all or some of these records will enable you to compile an accurate family health history that can be passed on to your descendants and given to your doctor to be included in your own medical history.

The genetic and familial diseases which should be included in your family health tree and which warrant additional research to document are:

- alcoholism
- allergies
- arthritis
- asthma
- blood diseases (hemophilia, sickle-cell disease and thalassemia)
- cancer (especially breast, bowel, colon, ovarian, skin and stomach, leukemia and lung)
- cardiovascular disease (high blood pressure, atherosclerosis, heart attack, hyperlipoproteinemia, stroke and congenital heart defects)
- congenital abnormalities at birth
- cystic fibrosis
- diabetes
- Down's syndrome
- dwarfism
- epilepsy
- hearing disorders
- Huntington's disease
- hypertension
- liver diseases (particularly hepatitis)
- mental illness (particularly manic-depressive disorders and schizophrenia)

- mental retardation (Down's syndrome or phenylketonuria)
- migraine headaches
- miscarriages
- multiple sclerosis
- muscular dystrophy
- myasthenia gravis
- obesity
- respiratory diseases (particularly emphysema, bacterial pneumonia and tuberculosis)
- Rh disease
- skin disorders (particularly psoriasis)
- sudden infant death (SIDS)
- suicide
- systemic lupus erythematosus
- Tay-Sachs disease
- thyroid disorders
- visual disorders (cataracts, dyslexia, glaucoma, retinitis pigmentosa)

Some medical terms that you might encounter in old records and their possible translations include:

- **Cholera infantum** — summer diarrhea of infants, which usually occurred the first summer after weaning from breast feeding.
- **Ague** — usually malaria, but could have been any fever accompanied by chills.
- **Milk leg** — thrombosis in femoral vein, often after childbirth; death from pulmonary embolism or pelvic infection (usual cause for milk leg).
- **Stomach trouble** — could be from complications of gastric ulcer perforation or pancreatitis, hemorrhage, or cancer.
- **Galloping consumption** — rapidly progressive tuberculosis.
- **Brain fever** — meningitis, encephalitis.

- **Throat distemper** — tonsillitis, diphtheria.

- **Malignant fever** — fever with hemolysis, malaria with hemorrhagic skin rash, meningococcal infection, putrid malignant fever or typhoid.

- **Softening of the brain** — dementia (syphilitic or nonsyphilitic), cerebral hemorrhage or stroke.

- **Bloody flux** — dysentery (etiology depends on area), shigella, salmonella, amoeba, typhoid, typhus, etc.

- **Putrid sore throat** — gangrenous pharyngitis, tonsillitis with peritonsillar or retropharyngeal abscess.

- **Rose cold** — hay fever (erroneously thought to be caused by rose pollen).

- **Creeping paralysis** — tabes dorsalis (syphilis).

- **A peripneumony** — pneumonia plus pleurisy.

- **Summer complaint** — diarrhea and vomiting (gastroenteritis).

- **Marasmus and dropsy of the brain** — hydrocephalus and wasting of the body.

- **Hemorrhage and inflammation** — ruptured aneurysm or swollen lymph nodes or superficial cancer with ulceration and bleeding; swollen lymph nodes from chronic infection such as tuberculosis, brucella, anthrax, straphylocossus, etc.

- **Dentition** — infantile convulsions, febrile seizures, infected dental cavities, mercury poisoning from teething powders.

- **Debility** — failure to thrive in infancy or old age, or loss of appetite and weight from undiagnosed tuberculosis or cancer.

- **Mortification** — gangrene, usually of the leg; trauma; infection; diabetes; aneurysm of the aorta.

- **Parisis (paralysis)** — probably from polio, stroke, or syphilis.

- **Eclampsia** — convulsions of any cause; later applied more specifically to those related to childbirth.

While researching your family tree you may encounter terms with which you are unfamiliar, and the spellings will vary considerably. Write them down exactly as you find them and then ask your family doctor or an internist to translate and explain them to you. Alternatively, by using a medical dictionary and a Latin dictionary you can translate many of the terms yourself. Or read an article entitled "Disease and Death in the Nineteenth Century: A Genealogical Perspective," by James Byars Carter, M.D. It appeared in the *National Genealogical Society Quarterly* in December 1988. This will provide you with a brief history of medicine, plus an outstanding glossary of medical terms found in old records.

7 — Using Personal Computers for Your Genetic Data

Genealogists were among the first consumers to discover the value of a personal computer. Several genealogical programs have hit the market in the past few years and most of them will allow you to enter genetic data about your ancestors. Even those programs that do not specifically mention this ability can be adjusted to include this field.

Even if you are not a genealogist, you can utilize a database management system to compile genetic data about your family. But for the genealogist, the use of a genealogical program and/or a database management system to compile genetic and health information about the family is an important new advance offered by this marvelous technology.

Basically computers are devices that make simple decisions rapidly. You will not find the word "maybe" in a computer's vocabulary, just plain "yes" and "no." By making millions of yes/no decisions per second, complex problems can be solved in rapid succession. The electronic components used to build the computer are called hardware, while the instructions that control the computer are called software.

Hardware

The heart of a computer is the central processing unit, or CPU for short. Whereas the CPU of the first computers filled cabinets, the CPU in a modern personal computer fits on an integrated circuit chip a fraction of an inch square. The CPU can perform simple manipulation of numbers such as addition, subtraction, and numeric comparisons. Multiplication, on the other hand, is not as easy for the CPU — it must add numbers over and over to simulate multiplication.

A computer stores data in its memory. Random Access Memory (RAM) stores data temporarily while the computer is running. When you turn the computer off, the data stored in RAM is lost. Disk storage, on the other hand, is permanent. Programs and data can be kept on a disk while the computer is off for later use. Data recorded on a disk will remain there until erased.

The third function a computer performs is the transfer of data to and from the outside. A keyboard and monitor permit interaction with programs running on the computer. Data from the computer is displayed on the monitor, while information can be typed into the computer through the keyboard. It is also possible to connect other devices such as printers and telephone modems to the computer for printing documents and sharing data.

Software

Computer hardware is the nuts and bolts of automatic processing, but equally important is computer software, which provides the detailed set of instructions for the CPU to follow. Software is to a computer what a tape or a record is to a stereo.

Several levels of software are used to achieve a desired result. At the lowest level, the operating system controls the flow of data throughout the computer. The IBM family of personal computers use DOS, which stands for Disk Operating System. A Disk Operating System includes the ability to pass data to and from a floppy or hard disk. At a higher level are application programs which accomplish a specific job. Examples of application programs include word processing and database programs. The disk operating system and application program work together to control the computer and produce the desired results.

Personal Computers

There is some debate over when personal computers were actually born. The January 1975 issue of *Popular Electronics* announced a "project breakthrough — the World's First Minicomputer Kit to Rival Commercial Models — the ALTAIR 8800." The ALTAIR 8800 was an immediate hit among pioneering hobbyists who bought the new computers as fast as they could be made.

However, some may argue that the first commercial personal computer was the Commodore Pet, which was indeed the first assembled, all-in-one, affordable computer. The Pet had a built-in monitor and keyboard as opposed to the ALTAIR which required the use of toggle switches and simple lights to access data.

The Pet was soon followed by the Apple II, bringing explosive growth to a company in a now classic story. Like the Pet, the Apple II had a built-in keyboard, but relied on a television set for displaying information. The Apple II had a much sleeker design than the Pet, and caught the imagination of thousands of new computer enthusiasts.

By the time the IBM Personal Computer was introduced in 1981 there were scores of other companies producing small computers. It wasn't long, however, before IBM dominated the market, creating a standard for hardware which is still the major force in personal computer design.

It is estimated that there are more than 13 million IBM or compatible computers currently in use. The successors to the Apple II have been joined at Apple by the Macintosh, which today is the most successful "non-IBM" personal computer.

Genealogical Computing is Born

Shortly after the first personal computers became available, programmers with an interest in genealogy realized how perfectly matched their interests were. Successful genealogy requires careful research, organization of information, and creation of reports — ideal tasks for a home computer. The first program to be offered to genealogists was called FAMILY RECORDS FILE SYSTEM, by L. J. Goree. The first issue of *Genealogical Computing*, published by Paul and Sara Andereck in July of 1981, contained two ads for commercial genealogy programs: ROOTS89 by COMMSOFT, and APPLEROOTS by CDS Corporation.

The early programs, although quite limited by today's standards, demonstrated how useful computers could be for genealogists. As a minimum, they provided ways to enter and edit information about individuals and families, search and organize data, and print standard genealogy charts such as pedigree charts and family group sheets.

SInce 1984 most genealogy software has been released for the IBM or compatible computers. There are more than a hundred programs available from various sources, approximately 10 percent of which are for the Macintosh or other non-IBM computers.

Genealogy Software for Genetic Analysis

Understanding the influences our ancestors may have had on us through inherited traits demands much more in the way of record keeping than simple charts. In addition to the history of events which can constitute a simple genealogy, information related to health, traits, and other genetic characteristics must be retained. With such information, trends and statistics can be computed. Genealogy charts that illustrate genetic threads can also be prepared to help analyze a family's genetic history.

To see how useful a computer program designed for genealogy can be for genetic analysis, it is helpful to take a detailed look at one which has been specifically designed to record and report data appropriate for such studies. ROOTS III, introduced by COMMSOFT in June of 1988, is available for the IBM and compatible computers. ROOTS III is the latest in COMMSOFT's series of genealogy programs which started in 1981 with ROOTS89.

ROOTS III is designed to store, retrieve and display information about individuals and families, including supporting data. Details for more than 65,000 individuals can be stored by the program. In addition to dates and places for important events, ROOTS III allows extensive source documentation to be stored for each event. Events for each person can be selected from a large list, or you can choose your own. There is much flexibility from person to person on what events can be stored.

Once data has been entered into the ROOTS III database, a large number of charts and reports can be printed. Family group sheets, pedigree charts and ahnentafel charts are among the standard forms provided. The program will also print formal reports using the "Record" or "Register" formats which are used in genealogical quarterlies. While you are printing, ROOTS III keeps track of names and the page numbers on which those names are found. When you are done, a table of contents and paginated index can be printed.

Entering Data

The data entry screen for an individual record is shown in the diagram on page 112. The fields provide for the person's name, occupation, up to six events, and links to the mother and/or father. ROOTS III builds all family connections from the simple link you establish between the mother and/or father and their child.

Flags — Along the right side of the edit screen are nine data fields called "flags." The flags can be used any way you wish to record special pieces of information. The legends for the flags can be defined to describe the data you wish to store. Each flag can be set to "yes" or "no" to signify whether or not that data applies. For example, if you wish to keep track of those people in your family who are twins, you can specify that one of the flags be labeled "twin." Each time you encounter a person in your family who is a twin you would set the corresponding flag to yes.

Flags can be used singly or in combination. In the twin example above, a single flag was used. Since there are nine flags for each person, and three flags for each marriage, it is also possible to assign combinations of flags. For instance, by using two flags it is possible to have four pieces of information represented. The table below illustrates how four pieces of information can be kept by two flags:

Family Diseases: Are You at Risk?

```
Record:      39                    Last edited on:   10 Mar 1988
Name: Caroline Bouvier Kennedy
 Sex: F  Ref: KENNCB57   Parent Code: N    Ancestor Interest: 0      *: N   ArlCem: N
 Occ:                     Birth Code: L   Descendant Interest: 2             HlyCem: N
              (Interest and sure flags: 0 = lowest, 3 = highest)            ActPol: N
Born: 27 Nov 1957 2 New York City, NY                                       HarUni: Y
 Res: _____ N _____                                  GraLau: Y
    : _____ N _____                                  PbBook: N
    : _____ N _____                                  HCrCem: N
    : _____ N _____                                  MrInfo: N
    : _____ N _____                                  FLAGS
      DATE    SURE                         PLACE                            1917-1963
Father: John Fitzgerald Kennedy                                            1929-
Mother: Jacqueline Lee Bouvier
RecFnt: 00005
Double Dating: From 1 Jan to 24 Mar, enter later year from 1583 to 1752
Press CHANGE to start or end surname

                                                    KENNEDY
f1 John Fitzgerald Kennedy                      M   12 Dec 1988
f2 Caroline Bouvier Kennedy                     F   1917 - 1963
f3                                                  1957 -
f4
f5
Fam|Trace|Kshp  Edit|S/M  Print  Vit|Loc|Ann|Name|Year|Rel|Mod|DFoot|Oth|Grpng
```

Data entry screen for record from Roots III

Fact	Flag A	Flag B
Fact 1	no	no
Fact 2	yes	no
Fact 3	no	yes
Fact 4	yes	yes

The ROOTS III flags are the best way to preserve genetic information because the search and report functions can be based on flags. For example, a list can be created containing all individuals who have a specified flag set. Using this list, detailed reports can be printed. A special ROOTS III report, described in detail later, will contain statistics based on flags.

Reference Field — Coded data can also be entered in the reference field available for each person in the database. The reference field is eight characters long and can be filled with upper case letters and numbers. It is possible to place direct information in the reference field, such as the word "TWIN," or coded information such as "ABC123ZZ." The contents of the reference field can be searched to create special lists for reporting, just as with flags.

Footnotes — Each event in the database can have its own footnote. The simplest footnote contains a text description of the event. For example, the cause of a person's death can be included in the "died" event for that person. If you are able to determine that an ancestor died from heart disease, that fact can be entered in the corresponding footnote. As with the reference field, the content of footnotes can be searched to create a list of people who had specific causes of death.

Retrieving Data

The ROOTS III search routines provide a powerful way to find people in the database. Eight search routines span the major data categories which can be used as the basis for a search. When individuals are found in one of the search routines, their names can be used for other ROOTS III functions, such as editing or printing.

The simplest search routine finds all people who have a specified name. Using the *Names* search routine it is possible to find all individuals in the database having a particular name, such as Kennedy. The search can be narrowed by asking for all those having the name John and Kennedy but not Fitzgerald. Likewise, places can be searched for individuals who may have an event recorded there. A typical request might be to find all individuals who have an event recorded in Boston.

The *Vitals* search routine is used to search for individuals who have specified flags set. The flag search can be combined in this function with the presence of events for that person. You can search for all individuals who have the "A" flag set to "yes" and who are deceased.

Reference field data can be searched in the *Names* search function. It is possible to locate everyone who has specific data in the reference field just as you might search for those who have specific names. If you had entered "TWIN" or "TRIPLET" in the reference field of people in your family, you could look for everyone who was a twin or a triplet.

The footnote data can also be searched to find people in the database who have specific information recorded in that field. If you have been systematic about including the cause of death in the "died" footnote, you can locate easily all people who died from a specific cause. To see a list of all people who died of heart disease, the *Detail/Major Footnote Search Database* function can be used by typing "HEART DISEASE" in the corresponding search window.

Subject Grouping — The power of the search database routines is increased by a ROOTS III function called *Grouping*. With this, the results of multiple searches can be collected in a list called the grouping table. The contents of the grouping table can be used to spawn new databases or to feed the print routines.

Each of the eight search database routines send names of individuals to the grouping table. If you use more than one search database routine, the combined results are sent to the grouping table. If you then print a heredity statistics chart, the statistics in the chart will be based on the individuals in the grouping table.

A simple example of grouping might be to find all individuals with a certain surname — Kennedy, for example — who have an event recorded in a specific place (such as Boston). Using *Names*, one would first isolate all individuals in the database with the surname Kennedy. Next, one would use locations to narrow the name list to those who have an event in Boston. The grouping table result would be a list of Kennedys who have an event in their lives in Boston.

The list can be narrowed further with other search routines, such as *Vitals*. Perhaps you want to find all Kennedys who had an event in Boston and who have their "A" flag set to "yes." If you have defined the "A" flag to mean "graduated from law school," the list will contain law school graduates. The heredity statistics chart will contain only statistics on family members with the name Kennedy who had an event in Boston and who graduated from law school.

Reporting Family Data

Heredity Statistics Chart — The heredity statistics chart is the most useful printed report created by ROOTS III for looking at family statistics. The first step in printing a heredity statistics chart is to specify the starting person. The program then looks for all ancestors of that person to derive statistical information. Only individuals in the grouping table are included in the search.

A sample heredity statistics chart is shown in the diagram on page 116. The chart results are separated into three groups: statistics for all male ancestors; all female ancestors; and the composite of male and female. The number of generations included in the search is shown immediately below the preparer.

For the three groups a number of statistics are computed: ages at christening, at first marriage, at birth of first child, at birth of last child,

```
┌─────────────────────────────────────────────────────────────────────────────┐
│   HEREDITY STATISTICS REPORT FOR CAROLINE KENNEDY        11 DEC 1988          │
├─────────────────────────────────────────────────────────────────────────────┤
│                                                                               │
│  Ancestors of;   Caroline Bouvier Kennedy                                     │
│                                                                               │
│  Prepared by:    Linda A. Holmes 2257 Old Middlefield Way, Mt. View, CA 94043 │
│                                                                               │
│  Generations:    8                        Flags yield: 100.0%                 │
│                                                                               │
│                             POP  MEAN  STD  MIN  MAX  UNITS  RECORD NUMBERS    │
│                                        DEV                    MIN      MAX     │
│  MALE ANCESTORS:     34                                                        │
│    Age at christening        2   0.0   0.0  0.0  0.0  years    1        1      │
│    Age at first marriage    10  28.5   4.8 21.4 37.1  years  155      180      │
│    Age at birth of first child 16 31.0 7.0 21.0 51.0 years  119      168      │
│    Age at birth of last child  16 33.9 8.3 21.0 51.0 years  119      168      │
│    Age at death             13  71.5  15.1 35.4 87.6  years   69      152      │
│    Number of marriages      30   1.0   0.0  1    1            4        4       │
│    Number of children       34   1.6   1.6  1    9          152        1       │
│                                                                               │
│  FEMALE ANCESTORS:    30                                                       │
│    Age at first marriage     9  24.2   3.0 21.0 29.9  years  151      120      │
│    Age at birth of first child 11 27.9 5.3 21.0 39.5 years  116      154      │
│    Age at birth of last child  11 33.2 7.2 21.0 41.5 years  116        2       │
│    Age at death              8  70.1  17.2 43.0 98.8  years  151      157      │
│    Number of marriages      30   1.1   0.3  1    2            2       37       │
│    Number of children       30   1.7   1.8  1    9          157        2       │
│                                                                               │
│  ALL ANCESTORS:     64                                                         │
│    Age at christening        2   0.0   0.0  0.0  0.0  years    1        1      │
│    Age at first marriage    19  26.5   4.2 21.0 37.1  years  151      180      │
│    Age at birth of first child 27 29.8 6.4 21.0 51.0 years  119      168      │
│    Age at birth of last child  27 33.6 7.9 21.0 51.0 years  119      168      │
│    Age at death             21  71.0  15.9 35.4 98.8  years   69      157      │
│    Number of marriages      60   1.0   0.2  1    2            4       37       │
│    Number of children       64   1.7   1.7  1    9          152        2       │
│    Age of all children at death  68 58.2 27.2 0.0 98.8 years   4      155      │
│    Age of non-infant children at death 64 61.8 23.9 1.2 98.8 years 80 155     │
│    Male children           108  47.2                  percent                 │
│    Female children         108  52.8                  percent                 │
│    Still births            108   1.9                  percent                 │
│    Multiple birth events    64   2.1                  percent                 │
│    Records with "ArlCem" flag set 64 1.6              percent                 │
│    Records with "HlyCem" flag set 64 1.6              percent                 │
│    Records with "ActPol" flag set 64 4.7              percent                 │
│    Records with "HarUni" flag set 64 3.1              percent                 │
│    Records with "GraLaw" flag set 64 1.6              percent                 │
│    Records with "PbBook" flag set 64 3.1              percent                 │
│    Records with "HCrCem" flag set 64 6.2              percent                 │
│    Records with "MrInfo" flag set 64 23.4             percent                 │
│                                                                               │
└─────────────────────────────────────────────────────────────────────────────┘
```

Heredity statistics chart from Roots III

and at death. Next are shown the number of marriages and children, and, optionally, the number of illegitimate ancestors and marriages ending in divorce or annulment. The composite data includes the ages of all (including non-infant) children at death, and the numbers of male, female, stillborn and multiple birth events.

Generally, there are four types of data shown for each statistic. "Population" specifies the number of individuals used in formulating the statistic. "Number of Years" specifies the age at which the particular event happened to the population. (The "Years" statistics have four additional values: mean, standard deviation, minimum and maximum.) "Count" is the number of events for the population, and "Percent" is the ratio of the number of events to the total population.

Flags can play an important role in the heredity statistics chart. Flags can be used to determine who will be included in the statistics, and percentages of occurrences for flags can be shown on the chart. When setting up the heredity statistics chart, one of the options allows you to select or deselect individuals based on flags. You can choose to include or exclude only those records which have a specific flag set to "yes." If you use a flag to designate cause of death, and exclude records based on that flag, then the statistics will apply only to those who did not die of that cause.

A second option is to have the heredity statistics chart show the percentage of occurrence of a given flag. Rather than excluding or including records when a flag has been set to "yes," the program will compute the ratio of the number of "yes" flags to the population expressed as a percentage. Using this capability you can see what percentage of a family branch may have died from a certain cause.

Even though statistical techniques are used to compute the data in the heredity statistics chart, it is extremely important not to take the numbers too seriously. Because of all the factors which change over time — lifestyles, environmental factors, medical advances, etc. — information from the chart should only be used as an indicator of what has happened in the past with your family.

Other Genealogical Charts — The heredity statistics chart described above can be used to look for characteristics and trends that may be genetically based. ROOTS III produces a wide range of additional charts, many of which will be more recognizable as traditional genealogical reports.

The pedigree chart traces family lines back in time, showing the expanding tree of ancestors in graphical form. It is possible to show the data entered in the reference field for each individual as the chart is printed. If you have used the reference field for data, it will be easy to spot where family characteristics may have originated.

The family group sheet contains data about the husband, wife, and children in a family unit. More detail is provided about the spouses since the report is centered on them. Reference field data and flag information can be included for the mother and father.

If you wish to compile a formal genealogy, ROOTS III provides "Record" and "Register" formats for printing descending or ascending genealogies. Once again, the flag data can be included in the report so that others will be able to follow trends and characteristics that may show a genetic connection.

Currently COMMSOFT has a new form of pedigree chart in development. This chart is produced by a pen plotter which uses colored pens. In addition to allowing many generations to be printed on one page, the pilot program can use different colors for a person's name if a flag has been set for that person. By using colors, possible genetic connections can be graphically displayed. The program uses a ROOTS III database for information, and can print up to twenty-five generations on one page.

Future Programs and Uses

Today's personal computers available for genealogical processing are much more powerful than the first commercial electronic computer used by the Census Bureau back in the 1950s. Furthermore, the size of computers has been dramatically reduced. What fits easily on a desktop today would have filled rooms yesterday. Given the improvements in speed, memory, and size in just a few short years, it is exciting to think what the future will bring.

As genealogical databases become larger and more complete, the sharing of information will play a larger part in research. Data interchange standards now in development will allow information from one database to be easily exchanged with another, helping build more detailed family histories. Through this improved flow of information we will be able to gain a better understanding of our past. Armed with such knowledge we are then in a better position to know and understand ourselves.

8 — Your Family Health Tree: A Legacy for Your Descendants

Once you have researched your family's medical history, the information needs to be put into some form that can be understood easily by your family, your physician and your descendants for years to come. While you may not be able to collect a complete account of your family's medical history, it is important that you compile what you learn and put it into the form that can be of greatest use.

Drawing Up a Pedigree

The form of greatest use is a pedigree, which for this purpose is a pictorial representation of the health history of a family. Pedigree information for the family health tree falls into two categories. One is composed of basic data, which includes name, age, and ethnic origin, with family members represented by symbols and arranged in the correct place upon the family tree. The other is composed of the relevant medical information about each person.

The common pedigree symbols used are illustrated on page 69. These common symbols are used internationally and will be recognized by genealogists, physicians and geneticists. Males are represented by squares and females by circles. Sibling relationships are recorded in age order, if possible. Members of the same generation appear on the same line and branched bars attach siblings.

Medical pedigrees usually begin with the proband, which is a genetic term for an affected family member. However, your medical pedigree can begin with you or your spouse, in which case use an arrow to designate the proband as the central person around whom the medical pedigree is constructed. Or you may simply want to record on this chart all the known (or likely) genetic disorders that you find. All brothers and sisters are recorded in chronological order, including any deceased siblings and additional pregnancies, to reflect critical information concerning stillbirths, miscarriages or spontaneous abortions. The maiden names of all females are used.

It is important to designate half and/or full brothers and sisters in order to clarify relationships. Adopted children are identified with a broken line, since they are not biologically significant in a pedigree.

Now you have the symbols and your data, you are ready to construct the medical pedigree. First be sure that you have acquired all the information you need, i.e. names, ages, deaths and ethnicity. The reason ethnicity is important is that it can warn you to look for genetically inherited diseases that are more prevalent in particular populations. For example, Tay-Sachs disease is common in Jewish populations, cystic fibrosis in Caucasians, sickle-cell disease in blacks and neural tube defects (spina bifida) in people of Irish descent.

Quite likely you will discover that you are missing some information on certain family members, or you may discover there is a genetically linked disorder in your family that makes additional research necessary. Probably you will have to do several rough drafts of your medical pedigree before it is complete.

Asking the Right Questions

It is common to concentrate on the major health problems and to make many erroneous assumptions. It will help to ask the right questions. Some questions that are often overlooked of the mothers are: "Are these all of the pregnancies you have had?" and "Are these children all from your present marriage?" Categories that are often neglected include: mental illness, suicide, infertility, extreme tall or short stature, learning disabilities, speech problems and allergies. Other information that is often missed involves medical problems that were treated long ago and forgotten. Possibly family members had repaired hernias or surgery on cleft lip and palate, or there are unrecorded miscarriages and stillbirths; there may have been dental problems; and be sure to ask about any reconstructive surgery that family members may have had.

As a matter of fact, you will probably need to go back to family members a number of times to ask more specific questions. Often the original questions will be too broad and may require more details. At the end of this chapter there is a list of physical traits, characteristics and medical problems that you can use as a guide to extract more information about the family's medical pedigree. By giving a copy of this list to family members you may help to jog their memories about the family's health problems. Then you can ask such questions as, "Did Uncle John have any sight or hearing problems? Any unusual birthmarks or moles? Did he suffer from heart disease? Is there anything else that you can think of that gave him health problems? Did he ever have any surgery? What type? Why? Any emotional problems?"

Remember that unless all of your family members are medical doctors or geneticists, the information they provide may be faulty (and even experts are subject to errors) and the terminology may be incorrect. Write down the information exactly as given. However, verify it later with additional research. Aunt Julia may consider herself an expert on the causes of death of family members or about the illnesses of her loved ones, when in fact she may be woefully incorrect or could have mixed up her information. She may tell you, for example, that grandmother suffered from arthritis, when in fact it was grandpa.

Using this line of questioning you may discover information that was overlooked in the original interview with family members. So after you have constructed your first draft of the pedigree, obtained as much specific information as possible and recorded the documented data (from death certificates, hospital records, etc.), you should go back and ask general questions that cover the entire family.

Ask such things as: "Are there any other unusual traits or medical problems in family members, like cancer, alcoholism or drug addiction, emotional or mental illness, learning problems, seizures, surgeries, broken bones, extremely tall or short stature?" It is also a good idea to record the height of the immediate family members because extremely short or tall stature commonly occurs in many genetic, chromosomal or inherited disorders.

Another type of questioning is the open-ended kind such as: "Can you think of any traits running in our family that seem unusual?" Since all families exhibit certain traits that seem to be rare in other families (lip pits, ear tags, extra fingers, wide-spaced eyes, hollow chests, etc.), by asking this question you may discover that premature graying occurs or that family members have peculiar moles or birthmarks.

Getting All the Information

Once you learn about a certain illness or medical problem, probe for additional details. For example, if you discover a family member has diabetes, it is important to learn at what age it was diagnosed, how it was treated, and if there are other family members with diabetes. In the event you discover a cousin who is mentally retarded, find out as much information about the retardation as possible. How did it develop? Where was it diagnosed? Does he or she look different from other family members? How so? In such cases it is also wise to track down any available medical records, ask if any tests have been done and determine if any other health problems exist.

Occasionally in your research you may discover things which on the surface do not appear to be genetically related — such as a family member who had numerous broken bones, supposedly caused by accidents. While that may well be the case, it should not be taken for granted, since certain groups of genetically inherited bone disorders show up in the tendency to frequent breaks. If possible obtain all information about deaths in the family — the cause and circumstances and the age of the individual. Suicides may be the result of mental illness, environmental stress, or knowledge of a fatal illness such as Huntington's disease or cancer. These are sensitive areas to probe, but can be handled with delicacy and concern.

Sometimes there is hidden information in what appears to be ordinary material. For example, your grandmother may tell you she had a brother who was deaf but neglect to tell you that his deafness was caused by a childhood accident, which would eliminate a genetic cause. However, since about 50 percent of deafness has a genetic component, it is important to learn the cause of that relative's deafness. If the deafness resulted from an accident or from rubella (German measles), then the family is at no risk of recurrence.

You should always ask about the reason for blindness (which is also 50-percent genetic), deafness, muscle weakness, surgery and mental retardation (which may be from an accident, infection or high fever rather than a chromosomal or genetic cause). If the cause is unknown or unclear simply record the descriptions of the trait or disorder as the person gives it to you and place a question mark after that information.

The rules that should guide you in collecting and compiling your family's medical pedigree are:

1) Use standardized symbols for each pedigree and add the key to these symbols on each of your charts. This will help those who read it years later.
2) Use a specific set of medical questions. Use those found on pages 126-128 to ask questions of all family members.
3) Be as thorough as possible, recording all information even if you question the value of a particular piece of data. It may not seem important to you but may be very meaningful to your doctor or to a geneticist. Also get as much information as possible about each trait or condition you encounter when you interview family members.

Constructing a Medical History Chart

Medical pedigrees like the one on page 124, which shows four generations, are normally used to show a particular type of disease or disorder and how it occurs in a particular family. To get an overview of what your family's medical history looks like, construct a chart, beginning with your great-grandparents, if known, to show family members' ages at death and their major health problems and causes of death.

This chart deals with your direct line, and it is an ideal chart to be included in every genealogy. It is often difficult to determine genetic disorders in a family without the aid of a geneticist, but for most purposes what is important is to record the various diseases that have plagued your family over the years. This can serve to alert family members to their predisposition toward certain health problems. You can do this by incorporating several kinds of charts or by preparing a simple family health record like the one on page 125, which can be expanded by adding the siblings of each couple's grandparents on a separate form. For genealogists who want to record all the medical and health data found about all their ancestors, it will probably be necessary to construct several pedigree charts or to use a computer to assemble and compile information.

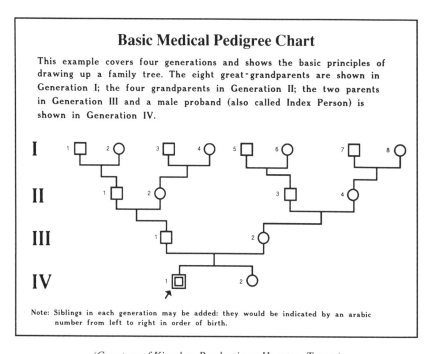

Basic Medical Pedigree Chart

This example covers four generations and shows the basic principles of drawing up a family tree. The eight great-grandparents are shown in Generation I; the four grandparents in Generation II; the two parents in Generation III and a male proband (also called Index Person) is shown in Generation IV.

I

II

III

IV

Note: Siblings in each generation may be added: they would be indicated by an arabic number from left to right in order of birth.

(Courtesy of Kingdom Productions, Houston, Texas.)

FAMILY HEALTH RECORD

NAME	BIRTH DATE	BLOOD TYPE & Rh	OCCUPATION	DISEASES & INFIRMITIES	IF DECEASED AGE & CAUSE
HUSBAND					
HIS FATHER					
HIS MOTHER					
HIS BROTHER OR SISTER					
HIS BROTHER OR SISTER					
HIS BROTHER OR SISTER					
HIS BROTHER OR SISTER					
HIS BROTHER OR SISTER					
HIS PATERNAL GRANDFATHER					
HIS PATERNAL GRANDMOTHER					
HIS MATERNAL GRANDFATHER					
HIS MATERNAL GRANDMOTHER					
WIFE					
HER FATHER					
HER MOTHER					
HER BROTHER OR SISTER					
HER BROTHER OR SISTER					
HER BROTHER OR SISTER					
HER BROTHER OR SISTER					
HER BROTHER OR SISTER					
HER PATERNAL GRANDFATHER					
HER PATERNAL GRANDMOTHER					
HER MATERNAL GRANDFATHER					
HER MATERNAL GRANDMOTHER					

Questions Checklist

Sensory Organs

Eyes

☐ blindness
☐ farsighted/nearsighted
☐ cataracts
☐ glaucoma
☐ retinal detachment/retinal problems
☐ thick glasses/eye surgery/eye patch
☐ color blindness/night blindness
☐ different colored eyes (e.g. one blue, one brown)

Ears

☐ unusual shape
☐ hearing loss — deafness/hard of hearing
☐ hearing aids

Nose

☐ absence of sense of smell

Hair/Skin/Teeth

☐ psoriasis/eczema
☐ birthmarks — pink, brown, white
☐ moles
☐ skin tags
☐ premature balding or graying
☐ white patch of hair
☐ extra/missing/misshapen teeth

Nerve/Muscle/Bone

☐ slow learners
☐ learning disabilities
☐ mental retardation
☐ seizures/convulsions/epilepsy/fits
☐ fainting spells/dizziness
☐ mental illness — depression/schizophrenia
☐ speech difficulties
☐ migraine headaches
☐ shaking/twitching
☐ weakness
☐ dystrophy
☐ back problems
☐ bone brittleness
☐ clubfeet
☐ dislocated hips at birth
☐ tall/short stature
☐ pilonidal cysts
☐ loose joints
☐ double jointed
☐ arthritis

Respiration

☐ allergies/asthma/sinus/emphysema
☐ cystic fibrosis

Digestion/Metabolism

☐ ulcer/colitis
☐ high cholesterol
☐ gall bladder problems
☐ restricted diet
☐ thyroid/goiter
☐ diabetes

Reproduction/Excretion

- ☐ bladder/kidney infections
- ☐ variation in size/number of kidneys
- ☐ prostate problems
- ☐ undescended testicles
- ☐ infertility
- ☐ unusual reproductive organs (internal and external)
- ☐ hemorrhoids

Circulation

- ☐ heart murmurs
- ☐ varicose veins
- ☐ clotting
- ☐ bleeding disorders/hemophilia
- ☐ anemias
- ☐ high blood pressure/hypertension

Other

- ☐ cysts/lumps/growths/tumors
- ☐ extra fingers/toes
- ☐ webbing — fingers/toes
- ☐ hole in heart/congenital heart defects
- ☐ open spine/spina bifida
- ☐ hydrocephalus/waterhead
- ☐ surgeries
- ☐ serious illnesses
- ☐ cancer/leukemia
- ☐ alcoholism/drug abuse
- ☐ hernia
- ☐ numbness

9 — Genetic Counseling: Should You Consider It?

Genetic counseling is a relatively new scientific specialty that has expanded swiftly in recent years. It provides and interprets medical information based on increasing knowledge of human genetics, the branch of science concerned with heredity. The genetic counselor's major goal is to impart understanding of birth defects and genetic mechanisms to affected families, and to help prospective parents make informed decisions about childbearing.

Genetic counseling is concerned with all factors causing birth defects. Birth defects occur in more than 7 percent of all births today, with the number of affected families well in the millions. Each year, more than 250,000 American babies are born with physical or mental defects of varying severity. Some of these defects, though present at birth, do not become apparent until months or years later.

Those most often seeking genetic counseling are mothers age thirty-five or older, because the risk of having babies with certain chromosome defects increases as women reach their thirties and forties. The risk is the same whether it is the first child of an older mother or one of several. Others seek genetic counseling because they have already had a child with a birth defect, or because other family members have an abnormality suspected of being hereditary. Couples from ethnic groups at high risk of specific genetic disease also look for further information. However, many people who need the kind of help that genetic counseling provides fail to receive it, partly because they are unaware of its existence.

A couple who plan to have children should seek genetic counseling if either of them has a disease with a genetic component or has produced an affected child, or the mother is thirty-five or older. If hereditary medical problems such as cystic fibrosis, hemophilia, Huntington's disease, muscular dystrophy, retinitis pigmentosa, sickle-cell anemia, Tay-Sachs disease or Cooley's anemia have occurred in your family, and you plan to have children, you should consider genetic counseling and screening tests. Many couples are turning to genetic testing and counseling to see if they can conceive a healthy child.

What Genetic Counselors Do

Genetic counselors use as tools the basic laws governing heredity, plus knowledge of the frequency of specific birth defects in the population, to predict the probability of recurrence of a given abnormality in the same family. Sophisticated new techniques are being developed and refined that translate statistical estimates into accurate forecasts. Tests before pregnancy and before birth are used to determine the presence or absence of a growing list of inherited defects.

A genetic counselor must first determine whether the defect in question is transmitted by the genes passed from parents to children or is due to infection or other influences during life in the womb. Appropriate information can enable families and physicians to prevent defects or, in some cases, to reverse, or at least reduce, their damaging effects.

Before a family can be counseled, the nature of the birth defect in question must be established. Environmentally produced defects may mimic genetic disorders; differing genetic factors also can produce similar disease patterns; and a given hereditary illness can assume different forms in different patients. The geneticist begins by establishing a definitive diagnosis. The affected individual and sometimes others in the family must be examined. Sometimes they are given laboratory tests. Parents of an affected child will be asked for a family health history as complete as they can provide, perhaps two or more generations back.

When he or she is sure a given birth defect is present in a family, a genetic counselor may take special steps to identify other family members. For example, if one child of a couple has the metabolic disorder known as Wilson's disease (inability to excrete the copper found in most foods), other children in the family must be tested carefully for early signs of the same inherited defect. If these signs are found, prompt treatment can save them from serious liver and brain damage.

A family needing genetic counseling must first recognize the need. This may come through personal concern about recurrence of a condition within the family, or may be suggested by a doctor. In modern medical practice the importance of genetic disorders is being recognized by more and more family doctors. As a result, more patients are being referred to specialized counseling services.

When genetic studies are completed in a particular family, the counselor, the assisting health professional, or the referring physician to whom results are reported will not prescribe a particular course of action. The counselor's role is to provide the family seeking help with a realistic view of the situation — the nature of the birth defect already manifested in a family member, the risk of recurrence and what a recurrence would mean in practical terms for all concerned — and to assist affected families through a difficult time in their lives.

If there are decisions to be made — about care of the child already affected, about having more children, about the ability of the family to cope with ongoing problems — the parents can make more informed choices with the facts in hand. This includes information on community resources which can help them and their children.

Inherited disorders used to be accepted as flukes of nature about which nothing could be done. This is changing. Genetic screening identifies prospective parents at risk of having a baby with physical or mental problems. Doctors can diagnose hereditary disorders in early pregnancy as well as spot fetal and biochemical mistakes related to the mother's age, nutritional abnormalities or some other factor. Combined with genetic counseling, a prenatal diagnosis that reveals no problems can reassure worried couples. However, if a diagnosis turns up something amiss, it can be a timely signal to arrange for the birth in a hospital equipped to handle risky cases. But early warning of some problems poses a disturbing choice: if a fetus is diagnosed as having, say, Down's syndrome or some other serious flaw, there is the troubling question of whether to have the baby or terminate the pregnancy. This is a decision which only the parents can make. Many turn to their clergy or to support groups, which are becoming increasingly sophisticated in the field of human genetic problems.

Medical science can how diagnose at least 100 different birth defects. Many of them are rare, but some, such as Fragile X syndrome (a disorder causing mental retardation), occur more frequently than was once thought. If there is a hereditary disease in your family, or if you or a close relative has a child with birth defects, you should consider genetic screening.

Genetic counseling centers are often located in hospitals and clinics associated with medical schools. It is predicted that clinics and centers that test for genetic defects will multiply over the next few years. For now, though, extensive tests are performed mainly on pregnant women. A few leading medical centers also offer genetic tests for healthy adults whose family history indicates that they are at high risk of developing certain diseases at a later age.

What You Can Do

A genetic counselor will ask you to supply a detailed family history, as medically documented as possible. This will be in the form of a written questionnaire accompanied by a personal assessment. The counselor will address your concerns, summarize the risks, and state the alternatives. Deciding on what course to follow will be up to you, although your doctor probably will insist that you undergo certain tests if you are pregnant and your pregnancy appears to be vulnerable.

Genetic counseling can prepare you to cope, or it can ease your mind if no risk is found. However, it can raise some agonizing questions if a risk is found.

The older a pregnant woman is, the greater her risk of having a baby with Down's syndrome. Therefore, doctors usually suggest testing for its presence. Amniocentesis is the fetal test used most often to detect Down's syndrome and spinal abnormalities. It is also used to determine the stage of lung development in babies expected to be premature, and it can now detect some eighty additional disorders. If there is a history of chromosomal disorder in your family, or if you face a higher-than-normal risk of having babies with birth defects, your doctor will probably recommend that you have this test also, even if you are not yet thirty-five.

Those seeking genetic counseling are understandably apprehensive, for the information learned can affect their whole life — their concept of themselves and their dreams of having a family. There are several steps you can take to make the most of your visit to the counselor. First start thinking about genetics and your family's health history well in advance of the meeting. For a self-addressed stamped envelope, the March of Dimes will send you a helpful booklet entitled "Genetic Counseling" that explains genetic screening, and a worksheet called "Family Medical Record" for you to plot out the medical background of yourself, your spouse and various relatives. This will include questions relating to whether parents, grandparents or other close relatives had high blood pressure, undiagnosed paralysis, mental retardation or other diseases — all questions that a counselor will ask. (Call your local March of Dimes chapter or write to the March of Dimes Birth Defects Foundation, 1275 Mamaroneck Avenue, White Plains, NY 10605 to obtain this literature.)

Using this information, the counselor may ask you to undergo certain tests. At the meeting to discuss your family history and the test results, don't be afraid to ask questions. In a matter of such importance it is crucial that you understand everything that is discussed.

The point of counseling is to get information, not to make an on-the-spot decision as to whether you should have children or continue a current pregnancy. By consulting a counselor before a pregnancy you and your spouse can take the time to decide how that information will affect your childbearing plans. However, when you undergo a blood test or amniocentesis during a pregnancy and learn of a possible genetic defect in the fetus, you and your spouse are faced with the crisis of having to make an almost immediate decision about whether to have the child.

In such a case, the first step is to check the accuracy of the test — either by having it repeated or by having alternative tests for the same disorder performed. Not every test is 100-percent accurate, so it is important to exhaust all tests before making any decision.

If you and your spouse choose to have genetic testing done on yourselves or your developing fetus, you should be aware of the limits of such testing. At present, the science of genetics can only tell you if your child-to-be will suffer from particular genetic defects. It cannot tell you the extent of these defects or whether your child will or will not be able to cope with them. Many people with handicaps cope quite well and lead productive and rewarding lives. Even if testing does not indicate a problem, the baby may still be born with a defect or disease because not all deformities are genetic — and there are not yet tests for all genetic disorders.

Help for Family Members

Families whose members have genetic problems will need courage and help in order to adjust and to carry on their lives. Whenever a genetic disorder occurs in a family, particularly for the first time, it affects all family members, not just the parents or siblings living at home. Genetic disorders touch the extended family — grandparents, aunts, uncles and cousins — as well.

Professional and self-help groups sensitive to the needs of all family members are a valuable resource, for they can provide information and emotional support. At the end of this chapter is a list of mutual support groups concerned with the medical and psychosocial impacts of genetic disorders and birth defects on affected individuals and families. Each of the support groups is dedicated to serving the ongoing emotional, practical and financial needs of these populations. Through shared experience and understanding, these groups offer services and guidance crucial to the effective management of often frustrating and isolating situations.

Family members within the household need the most immediate support so they can learn as much as possible about the disorder and how to care for the affected person. Parents of a child with a genetic disorder are most likely to seek the services of self-help groups or professional counseling. They also may need guidance in dealing with the healthy child or children because often, due to the focus in many families on the genetic disorder itself or on the affected child, the normal child or children develop behavior problems.

Grandparents, aunts, uncles, cousins and close family friends will have different needs. They will be concerned about their loved ones and how they can help. But they will also want information about the genetic disorder, its frequency of incidence and the chance of carrying the defective gene across generations. They will also want to know what new research is going on for a particular disease (chapter 10 provides information about some of the genetic research findings and the research in progress). Sometimes family members are reluctant to ask such questions of the parents of the affected child and are more comfortable using professional or organizational sources familiar with the disorder. By contacting the appropriate organizations they can obtain the information and help they seek.

Regional Networks

Prior to 1978 genetic services were largely provided by university-affiliated teaching facilities scattered throughout the United States. With the funding that became available under the Genetic Services Act in that year, individual states were encouraged to develop statewide networks to improve the availability of genetic services to their own citizens. The Genetic Diseases Service Branch, Division of Maternal and Child Health, Department of Health and Human Services, began to provide funds for the states to organize into regional groups, or networks, with four objectives:

1) To assure good communication among adjoining states.

2) To collect data about services available within the region.

3) To work on quality assurance.

4) To provide education for the public and professionals about genetic diseases, the genetic services available, and the treatment and prevention of genetic diseases.

There are now genetics networks in almost every region in the country. The Council of Regional Networks is a group of individuals representing existing and planned regional genetic networks. Its aim is to provide a system for communication between genetic services regions and to serve as a forum for ideas relating to the public health components of medical genetics. The efficient use of scarce resources, the development of a common database, and a program of quality assurance are priority items for the group. The regional networks are as follows:

Southwestern Regional Genetics Network

California State Department of Health Services, Maternal and Child Health Branch, Genetic Disease Section, 2151 Berkeley, Annex 4, Berkeley, CA 94704. Telephone 540-2534.

Mountain States Regional Genetics Service Network

Colorado Department of Health, Family Health Service Division, 4210 East 11th Avenue, Denver, CO 80220. Telephone 303-331-8373.

Southeastern Regional Genetics Group (SERGG)

Emory University School of Medicine, Office of the Treasurer, Atlanta, GA 30322. Telephone 404-727-5840.

Midwest Regional Genetic Services Network (MRGSN)

Indiana State Board of Health, 1330 West Michigan St., Box 1964, Indianapolis, IN 46206-1964. Telephone 317-633-0805.

Great Plains Genetic Services Network (GPGSN)

The University of Iowa, Department of Pediatrics, Iowa City, IA 52242. Telephone 319-356-2647.

New England Regional Genetics Group (NERGG)

Children's Hospital Corporation, 300 Longwood Ave., Boston, MA 02115. Telephone 617-735-6109.

New York State Genetics Program

New York State Department of Health, Wadsworth Center for Laboratories and Research, Laboratory of Human Genetics, Albany, NY 12201. Telephone 518-474-6796.

Pacific Northwest Regional Genetics Network (PacNoRGN)

The Oregon Health Sciences University, Crippled Children's Division, 3181 Southwest Sam Jackson Park Road, Portland, OR 97201. Telephone 503-225-8342.

Mid-Atlantic Regional Human Genetics Network (MARHGN)

St. Christopher's Hospital for Children, Genetics Department, Fifth and Lehigh Avenues, Philadelphia, PA 19133. Telephone 215-427-5289.

Other Sources of Help and Information

National Organizations

Alliance of Genetics Support Groups, 38th and R Streets, N.W., Washington, DC 20057.

National Organization for Rare Disorders, P.O.Box 8923, New Fairfield, CT 06812.

National Information Resources

National Center for Education in Maternal and Child Health (NCEMCH), 38th and R Streets, N.W., Washington, DC 20057.

National Information Center for Orphan Drugs and Rare Diseases (NICODARD), ODPHP/NHIC, P.O. Box 1133, Washington, DC 20013-1133.

National Health Information Clearinghouse (NHIC), P.O. Box 1133, Washington, DC 20013-1133.

American Association of University Affiliated Programs (AAUAP), 8605 Cameron St., Suite 406, Silver Spring, MD 20910.

Publications of Interest

Comprehensive Clinical Genetic Service Centers: A National Directory. National Center for Education in Maternal and Child Health, 38th and R Streets, N.W., Washington, DC 20057.

International Directory of Genetic Services, by Henry T. Lynch, M.D., et al. March of Dimes Birth Defects Foundation, 1275 Mamaroneck Ave., White Plains, NY 10605.

Reaching Out: A Directory of Voluntary Organizations in Maternal and Child Health. National Center for Education in Maternal and Child Health.

A Reader's Guide for Parents of Children with Mental, Physical, or Emotional Disabilities, by Cory Moore, et al. National Center for Education in Maternal and Child Health.

National Genetic Voluntary Organizations

The following information about specific genetic voluntary organizations was compiled from *A Guide to Selected National Genetic Voluntary Organizations*, published by the National Center for Education in Maternal and Child Health. The organizations are listed in alphabetical order to aid you in finding the one of interest to you and your family. Many will direct you to the local chapter or a regional chapter in your area; others will send you literature. All will explain what their particular organization does and refer you to the proper source in your area.

Acoustic Neuroma Association (ANA), P.O. Box 398, Carlisle, PA 17013. Support and information for those who face or have undergone acoustic neuroma removal and those experiencing cranial nerve defects.

Alzheimer's Disease and Related Disorders Association, Inc. (ADRDA), 70 East Lake St., Suite 600, Chicago, IL 60601.

American Brittle Bone Society (ABBS), 1256 Merrill Drive, Marshallton, West Chester, PA 19380. Provides information on the brittle bone diseases, osteogenesis imperfecta and osteoporosis.

American Cancer Society, Inc., 4 West 35th St., New York, NY 10011. Has more than 3,000 local units.

American Celiac Society, 45 Gifford Ave., Jersey City, NJ 07304. Provides education and information material on gluten-free diets and referral to a gluten intolerance group.

American Diabetes Association, 2 Park Ave., New York, NY 10016. Has 700 chapters in all fifty states and the District of Columbia.

American Foundation for the Blind, Inc. (AFB), 15 West 16th St., New York, NY 10011.

American Liver Foundation, 998 Pompton Ave., Cedar Grove, NJ 07009. Concerns itself with diseases of the liver, gall bladder and bile ducts.

American Lupus Society, 23751 Madison St., Torrance, CA 90505.

American Narcolepsy Association, P.O. Box 5846, Stanford, CA 94305. Attempts to solve the medical and psychosocial problems associated with narcolepsy and related sleep disorders.

American Porphyria Foundation, P.O. Box 11163, Montgomery, AL 36111. Deals with this group of rare blood disorders.

American Society for Deaf Children, 814 Thayer Ave., Silver Spring, MD 20910.

American Tuberous Sclerosis Association, Inc. (ATSA), P.O. Box 44, Rockland, MA 02370.

Arthritis Foundation, 1314 Spring St., N.W., Atlanta, GA 30309.

Association for Children with Down's Syndrome, Inc., 2616 Martin Ave., Bellmore, NY 11701.

Association for Glycogen Storage Disease, Box 896, Durant, IA 52747.

Association for Macular Disease, Inc., 210 East 64th St., New York, NY 10021.

Association for Neuro-Metabolic Disorders, 5223 Brookfield Lane, Sylvania, OH 43560. Serves those affected with medical conditions caused by disturbances in body chemistry.

Caring, Inc., P.O. Box 400, Milton, WA 98354. Provides various support materials for parents and professionals interested in health and welfare of persons with Down's syndrome.

Celiac-Sprue Association (CSA/USA), 2313 Rocklyn Drive, Suite 1, Des Moines, IA 50322. Provides material and dietary information about celiac-sprue and the gluten-free diet.

Charcot-Marie-Tooth (CMT) International, 34-B Bayview Drive, St. Catharines, Ontario, Canada L2N 4Y6. Helps those with CMT syndrome, also known as peroneal muscular atrophy, and provides a registry for researchers enabling them to locate individuals for analyses.

The Children's Association for Research on Mucolipidosis IV, 6 Concord Drive, Moncey, NY 10952.

The Children's Brain Diseases Foundation for Research, 350 Parnassus, Suite 900, San Francisco, CA 94117.

The Children's Liver Foundation, Inc., 155 Maplewood Ave., Maplewood, NJ 07040.

Cooley's Anemia Foundation, Inc., 105 East 22nd St., Suite 911, New York, NY 10010.

Cornelia de Lange Syndrome (CdLS) Foundation, Inc., 60 Dyer Ave., Collinsville, CT 06022.

Cystic Fibrosis (CF) Foundation, 6931 Arlington Road, Bethesda, MD 20814.

Cystinosis Foundation, Inc., 477 15th St., Suite 200, Oakland, CA 94612.

The Dysautonomia Foundation, Inc., 370 Lexington Ave., Room 1504, New York, NY 10017.

Dystonia Medical Research Foundation, 9615 Brighton Way, Suite 310, Beverly Hills, CA 90210.

Dystrophic Epidermolysis Bullosa Research Association of America, Inc. (D.E.B.R.A.), Kings County Medical Center, 451 Clarkson Ave., Bldg. E, 6th Floor, Room E6101, Brooklyn, NY 11203.

Ehlers Danlos National Foundation, P.O. Box 1212, Southgate, MI 48195. This foundation is interested in collecting family history records.

Epilepsy Foundation of America, 4351 Garden City Drive, Landover, MD 20785.

Familial Polyposis Registry, Department of Colorectal Surgery, Cleveland Clinic Foundation, Building A-111, 9500 Euclid Ave., Cleveland, OH 44106.

Families of S.M.A. (Spinal Muscular Atrophy), P.O. Box 1465, Highland Park, IL 60035. Promotes public awareness of Werdnig-Hoffmann disease, Kugelberg-Welander disease, benign congenital hypotonia, and Aran-Duchenne disease.

Families with Maple Syrup Urine Disease, 24806 SR 119, Goshen, IN 46526.

Foundation for the Study of Wilson's Disease, Inc., 5447 Palisade Ave., Bronx, NY 10471. Deals with Wilson's disease and related disorders of copper and metal metabolism.

The Fragile X Foundation, P.O. Box 300233, Denver, CO 80203. Deals with the Fragile X syndrome and other forms of X-linked mental retardation.

Freeman-Sheldon Parent Support Group, 1459 East Maple Hills Drive, Bountiful, UT 84010.

Friedreich's Ataxia Group in America, Inc., P.O. Box 11116, Oakland, CA 94611. A primary goal is to benefit persons with Friedreich's ataxia and their families.

The Gluten Intolerance Group of North America (GIG), P.O. Box 23053, Seattle, WA 98102-0353. Offers assistance and information to persons with celiac-sprue and to their families through publications and seminars and by funding research.

Guardians of Hydrocephalus Research Foundation, 2618 Avenue Z, Brooklyn, NY 11235.

The Hemochromatosis Research Foundation, Inc., P.O. Box 8569, Albany, NY 12208. Hemochromatosis is one of the most common genetic disorders (a disorder of iron metabolism in which iron accumulates in tissues) but is rarely diagnosed before clinically manifest or before death. The organ damage that results from the disease is reversible and preventable with early diagnosis and treatment. One of the Foundation's goals is to identify families with the disorder through screening.

Hereditary Disease Foundation, 606 Wilshire Blvd., Suite 504, Santa Monica, CA 90401.

Hereditary Hemorrhagic Telangiectasia Registry (HHTR) (Osler-Weber-Rendu syndrome), RFD 3, Pratt Corner, Amherst, MA 01022.

Human Growth Foundation (HGF), 4720 Montgomery Lane, Suite 909, Bethesda, MD 20814.

The Huntington's Disease Society of America, Inc., (HDSA), 140 West 22nd St., 6th Floor, New York, NY 10011.

Hydrocephalus Parent Support Group, 225 Dickinson St., H-893, San Diego, CA 92130. Deals with issues when a child is affected with hydrocephalus, spina bifida or a related condition. Social interaction between families is encouraged.

The Immune Deficiency Foundation (IDF), P.O. Box 586, Columbia, MD 21045.

International Cystic Fibrosis (Mucoviscidosis) Association (I.C.F.(M.)A.), 3567 East 49th St., Cleveland, OH 44105.

International Institute for Visually Impaired, 0-7, Inc., 1975 Rutgers, East Lansing, MI 48823. For pre-school visually impaired children.

International Joseph Diseases Foundation, Inc. (IJDF), P.O. Box 2550, Livermore, CA 94550. Services to those affected by or at-risk to inherit Joseph disease.

International Rett's Syndrome Association (IRSA), 8511 Rose Marie Dr., Fort Washington, MD 20744.

Iron Overload Diseases Association, Inc. (IOD), 224 Datura St., Suite 912, West Palm Beach, FL 33401.

Juvenile Diabetes Foundation (JDF) International, 60 Madison Ave., 4th Floor, New York, NY 10010.

Laurence-Moon-Biedl Syndrome (LMBS) Support Network, 122 Rolling Road, Lexington Park, MD 20653.

Leukemia Society of America, Inc., 733 Third Ave., New York, NY 10017.

Little People of America, Inc. (LPA), P. O. Box 633, San Bruno, CA 94066.

Lowe's Syndrome Association, 222 Lincoln St., West Lafayette, IN 47906.

The Lupus Foundation of America, Inc., 1717 Massachusetts Ave., N.W., Suite 203, Washington, DC 20036.

Malignant Hyperthermia Association of the United States (MHAUS), P.O. Box 3231, Darien, CT 06820.

March of Dimes Birth Defects Foundation, 1275 Mamaroneck Ave., White Plains, NY 10605.

Muscular Dystrophy Association (MDA), 810 Seventh Ave., New York, NY 10019.

Myasthenia Gravis Foundation, Inc. (MGF), 15 East 26th St., Suite 1603, New York, NY 10010.

Myoclonus Families United, 1564 East 34th St., Brooklyn, NY 11234.

National Amyotrophic Lateral Sclerosis (ALS) Foundation, Inc., 185 Madison Ave., New York, NY 10016. Deals with Lou Gehrig's disease.

National Association for the Craniofacially Handicapped, P.O. Box 11082, Chattanooga, TN 37401.

The National Association for Parents of the Visually Impaired, Inc. (NAPVI), P.O. Box 180806, Austin, TX 78718.

National Association for Sickle Cell Disease, Inc. (NASCD), 4221 Wilshire Blvd., Suite 360, Los Angeles, CA 90010-3503.

National Association for Visually Handicapped, 305 East 24th St., 17-C, New York, NY 10010.

National Association of Radiation Survivors (NARS), 78 El Camino Real, Berkeley, CA 94705. Supports research into late onset effects of exposure, including genetic defects.

National Ataxia Foundation, 600 Twelve Oaks Center, 15500 Wayzata Blvd., Wayzata, MN 55391. Hereditary spastic paraplegia, ataxia telangiectasia and Charcot-Marie-Tooth syndrome.

National Down's Syndrome Congress, 1800 Dempster St., Chicago, IL 60068.

National Down's Syndrome Society, 141 Fifth Ave., Suite 75, New York, NY 10010.

National Easter Seal Society, 2023 West Ogden Ave., Chicago, IL 60612.

National Foundation for Ectodermal Dysplasias (NFED), 108 North First St., Suite 311, Mascoutah, IL 62258.

The National Foundation for Jewish Genetic Diseases, 250 Park Ave., Suite 1000, New York, NY 10017. Genetic diseases affecting descendants of Eastern and Central European Jews: familial dysautonomia, torsion dystonia, Gaucher's disease and mucolipidosis IV.

National Fragile X Support Group, Route 8, Box 109, Bridgeton, NJ 08302.

National Gaucher Foundation (NGF), 1424 K St., N.W., 4th Floor, Washington, DC 20005.

The National Hemophilia Foundation (NHF), The Soho Building, 110 Greene St., Room 406, New York, NY 10002.

The National Hydrocephalus Foundation (NHF), Route 1, River Road, Box 210A, Joliet, IL 60436.

The National Ichthyosis Foundation, P.O. Box 252, Belmont, CA 94002.

National Information Center on Deafness, Gallaudet College, 800 Florida Ave., N.E., Washington, DC 20002.

National Kidney Foundation, Inc., 2 Park Ave., New York, NY 10016.

National Lupus Erythematosus Foundation, Inc., 5430 Van Nuys Blvd., Suite 206, Van Nuys, CA 91401.

National Lymphatic and Venous Diseases Foundation, Inc., P.O. Box 80, Cambridge, MA 02140.

National Marfan Foundation, 54 Irma Ave., Port Washington, NY 11050.

National Mucopolysaccharidoses (MPS) Society, Inc., 17 Kraemer St., Hicksville, NY 11801.

National Multiple Sclerosis Society, 205 East 42nd St., New York, NY 10017.

National Myoclonus Foundation, 845 Third Ave., 4th Floor, New York, NY 10022.

The National Neurofibromatosis Foundation, Inc. (NF), 141 Fifth Ave., Suite 7-S, New York, NY 10010.

National Organization for Albinism and Hypopigmentation (NOAH), 919 Walnut St., Room 400, Philadelphia, PA 19107.

National Organization for Rare Disorders, Inc. (NORD), P. O. Box 8923, New Fairfield, CT 06812.

National Scoliosis Foundation, Inc., P.O. Box 547, 93 Concord Ave., Belmont, MA 02178.

National Sickle Cell Clinics Foundation, Inc., P. O. Box 8095, Houston, TX 77288.

National Society for Children and Adults with Autism, 1234 Massachusetts Ave., N.W., Suite 1017, Washington, DC 20005-4599.

National Support Group for Arthrogryposis Multiplex Congenita (AVENUES), P.O. Box 5192, Sonora, CA 95370.

National Support Group for Exstrophy, 5075 Medhurst St., Solon, OH 44139.

The National Tay-Sachs and Allied Diseases Association, Inc. (NTSAD), 385 Elliot St., Newton, MA 02164.

National Tuberous Sclerosis Association, Inc. (NTSA), Box 612, Winfield, IL 60190.

The Organic Acidemia Association, 1532 S. 87th St., Kansas City, KS 66111. Deals with organic acidemias and related rare metabolic disorders.

Osteogenesis Imperfecta Foundation, Inc. (OIF), P.O. Box 838, Manchester, NH 03105.

The Paget's Disease Foundation, Inc. (PDF), P.O.Box 2772, Brooklyn, NY 11202.

Parents of Dwarfed Children, 11524 Colt Terrace, Silver Spring, MD 20902.

Parkinson's Disease Foundation, William Black Medical Research Building, Columbia-Presbyterian Medical Center, 640-650 West 168th St., New York, NY 10032.

Polycystic Kidney Research (PKR) Foundation, 20 West Ninth St., Kansas City, MO 64105.

Prader-Willi Syndrome Association (PWSA), 5515 Malibu Drive, Edina, MN 55436.

Prescription Parents, Inc., P.O. Box 426, Quincy, MA 02269. Directs its services to parents of children born with cleft lip and/or palate and to affected adults.

Progeria International Registry, Dept. of Human Genetics, 1050 Forest Hill Road, Staten Island, NY 10314.

RP Foundation Fighting Blindness, 1410 Mt. Royal Ave., Baltimore, MD 21217. Retinitis pigmentosa (RP) and allied inherited retinal degeneration — at centers throughout the U.S. and England.

The Scoliosis Association, Inc., P.O. Box 194, Manhasset, NY 11030.

Society for the Rehabilitation of the Facially Disfigured, Inc. (SFD), 550 First Ave., New York, NY 10016.

Spina Bifida Association of America (SBAA), 1700 Rockville Pike, Suite 540, Rockville, MD 20852.

Support Organization for Trisony 18/13 (SOFT), c/o Kris and Hal Holladay, 478 Terrace Lane, Tooele, UT 84074.

Tourette Syndrome Association, Inc. (TSA), 40-02 Bell Blvd., Bayside, NY 11361.

Trombocytopenia Absent Radius Syndrome Association (TARSA), 312 Sherwood Drive, RD1, Linwood, NJ 08221.

Turner's Syndrome Society, Administrative Studies Building #006, 4700 Keele St., York Univ., Downsview, Ontario, Canada M3J 1P3.

United Cerebral Palsy Associations, Inc. (UCPA), 66 East 34th St., New York, NY 10016.

United Leukodystrophy Foundation, Inc. (ULF), 2304 Highland Drive, Sycamore, IL 60178.

United Parkinson Foundation (UPF), 360 West Superior St., Chicago, IL 60610.

United Scleroderma Foundation, Inc. (USF), P.O. Box 350, Watsonville, CA 95077-0350.

Williams Syndrome Association, 16211 N. Greenfield Dr., Clein, TX 77379.

Wilson's Disease Association, P.O. Box 75324, Washington, DC 20013. For Wilson's or Menkes disease.

Xeroderma Pigmentosum Registry, c/o Dept. of Pathology, Room C-520, Medical Science Building, UMDNJ-New Jersey Medical School, 100 Bergen St., Newark, NJ 07103.

10 — Genetic Research in Progress

For the first time in history there is a realistic possibility that major medical breakthroughs within the next decade may correct, cure, or find new treatments for genetic disorders. This expectation provides hope to many millions of Americans whose lives are touched by one of the more than 3,000 hereditary conditions.

In a major advance toward human gene therapy, research scientists late in 1988 successfully transplanted new genes into animal cells at the precise locations of defective ones, and the heathy genes replaced or repaired the old. This research brightens the prospects for treating fatal hereditary illnesses such as sickle-cell anemia and cystic fibrosis at the genetic level. Once the technique is perfected, perhaps in the next five years, scientists will rely on the natural gene-healing mechanism — a phenomenon known as homologous recombinant DNA — to cure diseases that have afflicted mankind for millenniums.

Until recently, prenatal diagnosis by means of maternal serum alpha feto protein (MSAFP) testing, chorionic villus sampling (CVS), amniocentesis, etc., afforded no options for corrective treatment. Today, phrases like "gene therapy," "enzyme replacement therapy," "bone marrow transplants," and "genetic engineering" offer hope where no hope existed before.

An example of medical breakthroughs was shown on the PBS television series "The Infinite Voyage," in which an episode on frontiers in biology was aired nationally on June 1, 1988. In it, George McCoy, who has the genetic blood-clotting disorder hemophilia, became the first person to be treated experimentally with a synthetic, recombinant DNA-based, Factor VIII blood-clotting protein. The experimental treatment, carried out by physicians at the University of North Carolina at Chapel Hill, has been successful during its first year and the genetically engineered protein has so far been safe and therapeutic. A second year of study on an improved version of the protein is planned.

Genetics Institute, Hyland Laboratories, and Baxter Travenol collaborated in the development of the protein. The product was tested on mice for safety and on hemophiliac dogs for efficacy before the Food and Drug Administration approved the use of a human subject. They chose UNC-Chapel Hill as the pilot site for clinical trials in humans because of the university's long history of research and treatment in hemophilia.

In the late 1960s medical researchers developed a method of preparing freeze-dried concentrates of clotting proteins from human plasma. Since that time, freeze-dried concentrates have been used extensively to control bleeding in people with hemophilia. Although the concentrates have been effective, they also have had drawbacks. Recent advances in blood-processing technology have reduced risks, however, and safe, new blood products are becoming more widely available. PBS included the story of the experimental blood clotting protein in its series because researchers involved in the recombinant DNA project hope that the knowledge gained from this breakthrough will help lead to a better control or even, some day, a cure for hemophilia by means of gene therapy.

Road Map of the Human Gene System

U.S. scientists hope to create a detailed road map of the entire human gene system, which they hope will lead to improved diagnosis of hereditary diseases, the development of new drugs and a host of unforeseen benefits. There is great enthusiasm for the project. It would make possible the mapping of genes responsible for muscular dystrophy, neurofibromatosis and the genetic sequences related to manic depression. A high-resolution map showing every human gene has only recently become feasible with the development of specialized automated technologies. However, it is expensive and will require highly sophisticated computer programs, including a supercomputer.

Cystic Fibrosis

Cystic fibrosis is the most common fatal genetic disease in the United States. It occurs in approximately one out of every 2,000 births, and the gene is carried by an estimated one in every twenty Caucasians. Approximately 30,000 young people in America currently have CF, and about twelve million Americans unknowingly carry the cystic fibrosis gene. (The Cystic Fibrosis Foundation is on the brink of developing a screening program for the entire U.S. population which would allow us to identify these twelve million carriers.) Most people who have the CF gene don't know it and have no symptoms. Both parents must be carriers of the gene to have a child with cystic fibrosis because the CF gene is recessive.

There is no cure, so far. But after decades of research scientists are now making dramatic strides in their understanding of CF. Two major areas of CF research have captured scientists' interest. One of those areas is the search for the cystic fibrosis gene. Working to pinpoint the gene has been like looking for a needle in a haystack. However, recent advances have allowed scientists to identify segments of the DNA which are "candidates" for the CF gene, and researchers in London have isolated one likely candidate.

A search that began with looking through the body's billions of base pairs of DNA was narrowed to eliminate 99 percent of all genetic material. In April of 1987 a "candidate gene" on chromosome 7 was identified, and it is currently being tested to determine if this is indeed the CF gene. Finding the CF gene is a goal, but more importantly it provides a key to understanding what is going wrong in the CF cell. Simultaneously, scientists are studying the CF cell to determine how and why it functions differently from a normal cell. They are looking for the basic defect in the cell that causes the body to produce the characteristic thick mucus and salty sweat. Researchers believe that when they fully understand the CF gene's effect on the cell they will be able to develop successful treatments to cure the disease.

Tremendous advances in diagnosis and treatment have vastly improved the outlook for people with CF. In 1955, when the Cystic Fibrosis Foundation was established, few children with CF lived to attend elementary school. Today, more than half are living beyond their early twenties.

The Cystic Fibrosis Foundation has established a network of privately funded, multidisciplinary research centers — thirteen of them — located at major universities in the U.S. and Canada. These research centers are responsible for some of the recent major advances in CF research.

The Foundation's office is at 6931 Arlington Road, Bethesda, MD 20814. You can contact the CF chapter in your state for information on patient services, family support telephone networks, public education and fund-raising events. There are informational pamphlets available — for example: "The Genetics of CF," "What Everyone Should Know About CF," and "Your Child and CF." There is also a directory of CF chapters and centers and a handbook for parents with children with CF.

Huntington's Disease

Huntington's disease (Huntington's chorea) was described in the medical literature more than 100 years ago, yet decades later scientists still don't know how this gene, present from birth, wreaks such havoc. Indeed, practically every aspect of the disease remains unexplained.

Huntington's comes from an abnormal and as yet unidentified gene. Those who are unaware of their family histories are shocked to find themselves becoming disabled during their most productive years. Those who know it's in the family must wait decades to see if the disease will strike them. Some decide never to have children, because if a parent has the gene, each child has a fifty-fifty chance of inheriting it — and everybody who has the gene gets the disease. Most juvenile patients inherit the disease from their fathers; and even in the adult form, symptoms develop three years earlier on the average when the gene is passed on by the father rather than the mother. No one knows why. The gene does not reside on the chromosomes that determine sex.

The best hope for researchers lies in identifying the gene that causes Huntington's, analyzing the protein that it may direct cells to produce and figuring out what the protein does. Several research groups are working on these problems. Hopefully, some answers are likely within a few years.

In the meantime, research has yielded one piece of information, but its value is debatable. As a result of ground-breaking work in 1983 by Harvard molecular geneticist James Gusella and his colleagues, it is now possible to test some people at risk and to tell with 96 percent certainty whether they carry the Huntington's gene. However, if they do have it, no one can help them. There's no cure, and except for drugs that may relieve depression and control the chorea for a time, there is no effective treatment.

About 25,000 Americans have Huntington's disease, and 125,000 more are at risk. It is a late-onset, degenerative disease of the nervous system — like Alzheimer's, which also appears to be hereditary in at least some cases. If the studies that have made it possible to predict Huntington's disease fulfill their promise of identifying its cause too, they may, in addition, reveal something important about this other incurable brain disease, which afflicts 2.5 million Americans.

Huntington's disease is caused by a dominant gene; and though about half of the genetic diseases that afflict man are caused by dominant genes, they are not thoroughly understood. Through genetic research, Huntington's may become one of the few dominant disorders to be well characterized, and thus offer clues about the workings of other dominant genes.

In 1986 Johns Hopkins Hospital in Baltimore and the Massachusetts General Hospital in Boston began offering the Huntington's test to adults at risk. Surveys taken before the test became available indicated that between 60 and 80 percent of those at risk would want it. However, now that it's being offered, many seem to have backed down. At Hopkins, which notified 350 people at risk, only about 70 have signed up so far. Of the 1,500 at risk in New England, only 32 have gone in for preliminary counseling. People in their thirties often want to know if they have the gene to help them decide whether to have children, and others who already have families want the test because they are worried about their children.

It is a dilemma. Though many people who are at risk say they want this test to find out if they have the gene, genetic counselors say they really want to find out that they *don't* have it. But 50 percent of them do. Not everybody who wants the test gets it. Some of those at risk do not have enough living relatives to enable geneticists to trace the marker; others turn out not to need it because neurological examinations reveal that they already have the disease, and some who qualify change their minds after the initial counseling. So this test has good potential, but it can also be emotionally destructive.

A research roster for HD patients and families has been established at Indiana University in response to a recommendation of the Commission for the Control of Huntington's Disease and its Consequences. This roster is national in scope. Every effort is being made to enlist HD families in all areas of the U.S. and some other countries. The primary purpose of the roster is to facilitate research in HD, and roster families play a key role in this research. The majority of HD families are usually eager to be involved in scientific investigation. They realize that through research lies hope, and that the promise of research can only be realized with the active participation of HD families.

The kind of data being collected includes: pedigree information, involving a complete family history and demographic data; educational background, socio-economic level and occupational history; clinical history of patient; psychiatric history of patient and family members; intellectual functioning and any changes in cognitive abilities; social history, including barometers of social stress such as alcoholism, drug abuse, crime; history of treatment; history of genetic counseling; and history of other disorders, either physical or psychiatric.

For further information, call or write: HD Roster, Department of Medical Genetics, Indiana University School of Medicine, 1100 W. Michigan St., Indianapolis, IN 46223. (Telephone: 317-264-2241.)

Down's Syndrome

It has been discovered recently that some families have a hereditary characteristic that predisposes them to Down's syndrome. Much previous work has shown that the risk of Down's syndrome increases with the age of the mother, but the hereditary factor is unrelated to the mother's age. This discovery was made in certain Greek families, and geneticists are now investigating whether a predisposition to having a child with Down's syndrome appears in other ethnic groups.

Colon and Rectal Cancer

A genetic defect may be responsible for a large number of cases of colon and rectal cancers. This discovery could lead to improved diagnosis. Scientists compared cancerous material from the colon and rectum with normal tissue from similar sites and found that some genetic material was missing from chromosome 5 in at least 20 percent of the tumors.

In another study, researchers located the gene for familial adenomatous polyposis (FAP) on the same chromosome. FAP is found in certain families and is characterized by the formation of numerous polyps in the colon which frequently become malignant if not removed. On the basis of these two studies, scientists suggest that mutations in the FAP gene may be involved in both familial and nonfamilial forms of colorectal cancer. Further research should provide methods for prenatal and presymptomatic diagnosis of a predisposition to colorectal cancers.

Doctors now recommend that everyone over fifty periodically undergo routine internal examinations for colorectal disorders. If there were a blood test that could alert people that they carry a greater risk of developing colorectal cancer, it might motivate them to seek frequent checkups. Researchers speculate that some remedies may be fairly simple: a diet high in fiber and calcium, for example, may prevent or compensate for these genetic deficiencies.

Joseph Disease

Two genes, located on different chromosomes, are associated with Joseph disease, a fatal genetic disorder in which loss of specific brain cells leads to paralysis. The first gene, found on human chromosome 1, appears to cause the disease, which is inherited as a dominant disorder. A second gene, called the modifier gene, reduces the severity of, or even eliminates, Joseph disease in persons who are expected to develop the disease.

Manic Depression

Evidence is growing that, in some cases of manic depression, there is a gene near one tip of the X chromosome that predisposes its bearers to the disorder. Scientists recently used DNA-cutting enzymes to locate two genetic markers — one for color blindness, the other for a chemical deficiency that causes anemia — at the end of the long arm of the X chromosome. The markers occurred overwhelmingly among subjects with manic depression or related mood disorders.

Additionally, in a study at the Free University of Brussels, Belgium, researchers found another manic depression marker in the same area of the X chromosome. In 10 families, DNA was isolated from 89 individuals, 41 of whom had manic depression or severe depression. A genetic marker for a blood coagulation factor located near the color blindness and anemia markers occurred mainly among family members with the psychiatric disorder. The genetic link was emphasized by the fact that no fathers and sons shared mood disorders.

There is probably more than one gene involved in predisposing people in different populations to manic depression, scientists say. For instance, there is a genetic marker on chromosome 11, linked to manic depression among the Amish, but researchers suggest that the long arm of the X chromosome may hold special promise for tracking down a predisposing gene. "Banking of DNA samples from high-risk persons may lead to the isolation and sequencing of the [X-chromosome] gene responsible for manic-depressive illness," they say.

Retinoblastoma and Duchenne Muscular Dystrophy

Certain types of cancer seem to run in some families, and recently a group of Boston-area scientists announced that they had discovered a gene that normally blocks retinoblastoma, a rare and often hereditary eye cancer that develops in children. As early as the 1970s geneticists believed that genes that normally protect against the cancer serve as "off" switches, restraining cells from replicating ceaselessly and forming malignancies. If the switches are not inherited or are somehow disabled, say by radiation, chemicals or viruses, cancerous growth might start.

This recent find raises hopes that other genes may soon be found that inhibit the more common cancers of the lung, breast and colon. Once the origin of a disease is understood then work toward its prevention or cure can begin.

Both the retinoblastoma and Duchenne genes were located by comparing DNA strands from healthy and diseased cells. It was discovered that there are two genes in healthy people that protect against the eye cancer. People born with both of these genes intact can usually sustain damage to one without developing retinoblastoma, but those born with one damaged gene nearly always lose the other and develop the disease. Discovery of the genes, researchers predict, will soon result in accurate prenatal and childhood diagnostic tests for retinoblastoma. Eventually advances in gene therapy may even lead to a cure, perhaps through the use of a bioengineered virus that would ferry copies of the healthy gene to the cells of a retinoblastoma victim.

Advances in treatment of Duchenne muscular dystrophy may also come soon. At the present time, while there is no cure for Duchenne muscular dystrophy, supportive measures such as physical therapy and bracing can help to slow down some of the crippling symptoms of the disease and improve the quality of life for the patient and his family. In the Muscular Dystrophy Association's worldwide research programs, scientists continue to work intensively to find a cure or effective treatment for DMD. In the meantime, genetic counseling can help families at risk to understand and deal with the decisions they must make.

For additional information and pamphlets, contact your local office of the Muscular Dystrophy Association. Its headquarters are located at 810 Seventh Ave., New York, NY 10019.

Breast Cancer

Breast cancer strikes about one in thirteen women in the United States. Among women who have had breast cancer surgery, those with extra

copies of a gene that is believed to be involved in the cancer process —
called an oncogene — appear to have an increased chance of recurrence,
according to a new study. Knowing who is likely to develop metastases
(the transfer of the disease to another part of the body) would allow
doctors to undertake preventive chemotherapy in only those people who
need it. Research is continuing in this oncogene theory of cancer
development.

Cleft Palate

Another study that could be a research springboard into the broad
arena of genetic disorders has been completed by research groups in
London, in Cambridge, Massachusetts, and in Reykjavik, Iceland.
Scientists report that they have localized the gene mutation causing cleft
palate. The genetic defect, studied in a large family in Iceland, appears
to be linked to the X chromosome, they say. Because cleft palate
develops during the stage of embryo growth associated with disorders
like spina bifida, closer analysis of the newly identified gene mutation
may elucidate the mechanism of other developmental abnormalities.

Lung Cancer

In October of 1987 scientists announced that they had identified the
genetic origins of small-cell lung cancer — a particularly deadly form of
lung cancer. They still do not know what causes the genetic defect that
leads to the disease, but researchers who discovered the link say cigarette
smoking is a candidate. The research points to a missing pair of genes
on chromosome 3 as the cause of the cancer. The mapping of such genes
is the first step toward identifying the biological product for which they
code, and may in turn lead to improved diagnosis and treatment of the
disease they normally prevent. Small-cell lung cancer accounts for about
20 percent of the 30,000 to 40,000 new cases of lung cancer that appear
in the United States each year. Overall, lung cancer is the country's
leading cause of cancer death.

Gaucher's Disease

Scientists have recently located a rare gene defect that often leads to a potentially fatal enzyme deficiency in infants; they have tracked the mutation to a site on chromosome 1. This finding will improve genetic counseling for victims of the most serious forms of Gaucher's disease, which is caused by the enzyme deficiency. The enzyme in question, glucocerebrosidase, breaks down a critical fat in certain body tissues. When this builds up, it can cause several types of Gaucher's disease. Type 1, the most common form, is characterized by an enlarged spleen and liver and by bone deterioration. The genetic mutation for Type I is carried by one in 600 Jews of Eastern European ancestry. Type II kills infants by about 2 1/2 years of age. In Type III, nonfatal neurological symptoms, including epilepsy, dementia and difficulty in controlling eye movements, begin during adolescence. Most of the estimated 10,000 to 20,000 people in the United States with Gaucher's disease have relatively mild cases of Type I. About 2 percent have Types II or III.

Work is under way on the development of a gene therapy to treat Gaucher's disease.

Alcoholism

It has been determined through twin, family and adoption studies performed during the last twenty-five years that alcoholism has major genetic determinants. However, the precise quantitative significance of these genetic determinants is still in question, as is their mode of transmission between generations. Answers to these questions could lead to rational strategies for prevention and treatment based on an understanding of how innate traits interact with the environment to produce alcoholism, according to David Goldman, M.D., in an article in *Alcohol Health & Research World* (winter 1987/88).

For information on alcoholism and the research on genetic predisposition to it you can obtain a free copy of "Alcoholism: An Inherited Disease" from the National Clearinghouse for Alcohol and Drug Information (NCADI), P.O. Box 2345, Rockville, MD 20852. This booklet provides a historical overview and discusses significant research on genetic predisposition to alcoholism.

Another helpful booklet is also available free from NCADI. It is entitled "Alcohol and Ethnic Minorities." It presents current information on the alcohol problems of Asian/Pacific Islanders, blacks, Native Americans and Hispanics.

NCADI also publishes the quarterly *Alcohol Health & Research World*. It contains current research findings and is available from the Superintendent of Documents, Government Printing Office, Washington, DC 20402-9371.

Rett's Syndrome

Rett's syndrome is a disorder that to date has been found to occur only in girls. Extensive laboratory investigations have not revealed a cause for Rett's syndrome, but there is a suggestion that since the syndrome is confined to girls, a genetic basis involving the X chromosomes may be indicated. The International Rett's Syndrome Association publishes a quarterly newsletter which keeps parents informed of current research in the field. It is a voluntary, non-profit organization whose aims are to provide direct support to other parents and to promote an awareness of the syndrome. Its address is 8511 Rose Marie Drive, Fort Washington, MD 20744.

Tay-Sachs and Allied Diseases

Tay-Sachs disease (TSD) is a fatal genetic disorder in children that causes the progressive destruction of the central nervous system. To date, there is no cure for TSD. However, there is active research being done in the United States, Europe and South Africa. Enzyme replacement therapy has been explored, and although it is a promising approach scientists still face serious obstacles.

The National Tay-Sachs and Allied Diseases Association (NTSAD) was founded in 1958 by concerned parents committed to the eradication of Tay-Sachs and allied diseases. NTSAD, through its programs of public and professional education, as well as its prevention services, testing and research, insures that the vast and critical needs of so many are not left unmet. A major thrust of NTSAD continues to be the promotion of TSD genetic screening programs through affiliated hospitals and medical centers. There are more than 100 hospitals and clinics nationwide that offer testing on an "ongoing" basis. As of 1988, more than 600,000 individuals had been screened for Tay-Sachs disease. Thousands of carriers have been identified, and hundreds of couples have been shown to be at "high-risk" (that is, each partner was identified as a carrier).

The ultimate goal of Tay-Sachs disease testing extends beyond mass population screening. Increasingly a vital aspect of family planning includes the awareness and knowledge of one's genetic profile. Carrier detection enables young people who may be vulnerable to plan for healthy families.

Booklets available from NTSAD include: "What Every Family Should Know" and "Services to Families." For these and for additional information on a testing program near you or on any other relevant program, call or write: The National Tay-Sachs and Allied Diseases Association, Inc., 385 Elliot St., Newton, MA 02164 (telephone 617-964-5508).

Polycystic Kidney Disease

Research is being conducted in experimental animal models and in patients on several aspects of this disease. The National Kidney Foundation, Inc., is the major voluntary health agency seeking the total answer to diseases of the kidney and urinary tract — prevention, treatment and cure. The National Kidney Foundation, Inc., is located at 2 Park Avenue, New York, NY 10016.

Thalassemia (Cooley's Anemia)

Scientific research on Cooley's anemia and similar genetic diseases is sponsored by the National Heart, Lung, and Blood Institute, the

National Institute of Arthritis, Metabolism and Digestive Diseases, the National Institute of General Medical Sciences and other National Institutes of Health, as well as by a number of voluntary organizations. Important in basic research are studies of the genes and how they function. Current clinical research is concerned with improving techniques for transfusion therapy, iron chelation therapy and prenatal diagnosis. Other needs are for a simple, dependable screening test for the thalassemia trait, and for easy and efficient ways to do screening and counseling.

Research is now being done on the possibility of using bone marrow transplantation in the treatment of Cooley's anemia. Studies in this area are now restricted to the use of experimental animals. However, it is possible that this form of treatment will be attempted for patients on an experimental basis in the future.

The Cooley's Anemia Foundation, Inc., 105 East 22nd St., New York, NY 10010 was formed by the parents of thalassemia patients in the United States. The aim of the Foundation is to help affected families keep in touch with each other, to raise funds to support research, to improve treatment facilities and to encourage blood testing and counseling and screening programs. Contact the Foundation for additional information.

Arthritis

The search for causes of arthritis has come a long way in recent years. Scientists have known for some time that certain people have a genetic susceptibility to arthritis, but genes are not the whole story. Today's scientists have specific clues to provide direction for their work, and more basic scientific knowledge about the causes of arthritis will be a stepping stone to better treatments and possibly even preventions.

The two areas that have shown the most promise so far in terms of prevention are osteoarthritis and osteoporosis. Osteoarthritis, the most prevalent form, affects almost 16 million people in this country. It is thought that one reason some people develop osteoarthritis is because the joints get more punishment than they can take. Scientists have observed that people with osteoarthritis of the knee have a greater history of knee injuries than does the general population. This suggests that injuries may play a role in eventually leading to this form of arthritis. Excess weight appears to be an important risk factor also.

Some of the most exciting findings in the area of osteoporosis prevention are in the use of estrogen therapy for women after menopause. Hormone replacement has been found to help prevent the acceleration of bone loss in post-menopausal women and is now recommended for women at high risk of developing the condition.

The science of the future in this area is molecular biology, which examines the molecules that regulate all body processes at the most fundamental level. Applied to arthritis, it can open the door to understanding the malfunction inside certain cells in the body which cause some forms of arthritis.

Scientists are now looking at the possibility of curing a wide range of genetic diseases with gene replacement therapy — replacing abnormal genes in cells with normal ones. A lesser-known rheumatic disease, the Lesch-Nyhan syndrome, will probably be one of the initial disorders in which gene transfer therapy in humans will be attempted. Because of this condition's relationship to other kinds of arthritis, investigating it may lead to answers for a variety of others. (The Lesch-Nyhan syndrome is a rare and fatal disease that includes features of gout and severe neurologic disorder.)

Since there is not yet a cure for arthritis, funding research is a high priority for the Arthritis Foundation. Scientists are concentrating on three main areas of arthritis research: (1) genetic markers; (2) the immune system; (3) infectious triggers.

Information and referral services are provided through a variety of brochures. Contact your nearest Arthritis Foundation chapter — there are seventy-one chapters nationwide — or the Arthritis Foundation, 1314 Spring St., N.W., Atlanta, GA 30309. Several brochures are available that pertain to types of arthritis, treatments and general information. Most of them are free.

Hereditary Ataxia

The National Ataxia Foundation (NAF), incorporated in Minnesota in 1957, has four goals: service, education, research and prevention. This foundation attempts to locate people and families with hereditary ataxia in order to provide them with information about this disorder. NAF can direct people to local resources which are designed to help meet needs such as medical diagnostic services, genetic counseling, family planning services, insurance, where to look for homemaker services, day activity centers and nursing homes.

One of the most crucial elements in the fight against hereditary ataxia is the development of patient and family awareness and the dissemination of accurate information to researchers, physicians and allied health professionals. NAF provides educational materials and information. This is done on a "direct request" basis through the NAF office and by periodic mailings, meetings and seminars.

NAF encourages and promotes research on the hereditary ataxias. This is done by NAF granting funds for new research projects which have the potential of expanding into major, multidisciplinary research programs supported by government or private agencies.

Without a medical cure, the only way to halt the spread of hereditary ataxia is for those who have the disease to decide on their own not to have children. For those individuals who have a genetic risk of developing the disease, a decision to delay having children until they have passed the expected age of onset would also stop the spread of hereditary ataxia. Genetic counseling can allow individuals and families to make their life decisions based on accurate knowledge and understanding, rather than on misinformation or half truths. The national headquarters of NAF is 600 Twelve Oaks Center, 15500 Wayzata Blvd., Wayzata, MN 55391.

Genetic research offers hopes for millions of families afflicted with genetic disorders and these recent breakthroughs provide rays of hope that scientists soon will find cures and treatments for diseases that have plagued families for generations.

Glossary

alleles — alternative forms of a gene, occupying a specific site on a chromosome, which determine alternative characteristics in inheritance.

amniocentesis — a method of prenatal diagnosis that involves withdrawal of a small amount of fluid from the amniotic sac that surrounds the fetus; the fluid contains cells shed by the fetus which can be analyzed.

autosome — any of the non-sex chromosomes; normal humans have 22 pairs.

carrier of genetic disease — a person who possesses a defective recessive gene together with its normal allele. The gene can be transmitted to progeny who will have the genetic disease if another copy of the recessive gene is inherited from the other parent.

cholesterol — a fatty substance found in all animal tissue.

chromosome — a rod-like structure found in the cell nucleus and containing the genes. Chromosomes are composed of DNA and proteins.

DNA (deoxyribonucleic acid) — the substance of heredity; a large molecule which carries the genetic information necessary for the replication of cells and for the production of proteins.

dominant — refers to a characteristic that is apparent even when the gene for it is inherited from only one parent.

dominant gene — a gene whose characteristic is apparent even when its allele on the paired chromosome is different.

enzyme — a protein which speeds up or catalyzes a specific chemical reaction.

gene — a unit of heredity; a segment of the DNA molecule containing the code for a specific function.

gene cloning — isolating a gene and making many copies of it by inserting it into cells and allowing it to multiply.

gene mapping — determining the relative locations of different genes on chromosomes.

gene splicing — joining pieces of DNA from different sources by using recombinant DNA technology.

gene therapy — the introduction of a normal, functioning gene into a cell in which that gene is defective.

genetic code — the "language" in which DNA's instructions are "written."

genetic engineering — altering genetic material to study genetic processes and potentially to correct genetic defects. *See also* recombinant DNA technology.

genetics — the scientific study of heredity — how particular qualities or traits are transmitted from parents to offspring.

genome — the total genetic endowment packaged in the chromosomes; a normal human genome consists of 46 chromosomes.

lipoproteins — compounds consisting of lipids (fatty substances such as cholesterol) and proteins.

marker — a detectable genetic variant, such as one of the ABO blood types. Some markers are found only among the victims of certain diseases and can be used to determine the presence of these diseases.

medical genetics — the study of the causes, symptoms, treatment and prevention of genetic disorders.

molecular genetics — the study of genetic mechanisms at the level of the DNA and RNA molecules and their components.

mutation — a change in the number, arrangement or molecular sequence of a gene.

nucleic acids — DNA and RNA, the molecules that carry genetic information.

oncogenes — genes that may play a key role in the development of cancer.

phenotype — the entire expressed physical, biochemical and physiological constitution of an individual, resulting from the interaction of the genetic endowment with the environment.

RNA (ribonucleic acid) — an essential component of all cells.

recessive — refers to a characteristic that is apparent only when genes for it are inherited from both parents.

recessive gene — a gene whose product is detectable only when its allele on the paired chromosome is the same.

recombinant DNA — the hybrid DNA produced in the laboratory by joining pieces of DNA from different sources.

recombinant DNA technology — techniques for cutting apart and splicing together pieces of DNA from different sources.

sex chromosome — one of the chromosomes (X or Y) involved in sex determination. Normal human females have two X chromosomes in each cell, while normal males have one X and one Y.

X chromosome — a sex chromosome. *See also* sex chromosome.

X-linked — refers to any gene found on the X chromosome or to traits determined by such genes. Refers also to the specific mode of inheritance of such genes.

Y chromosome — a sex chromosome. *See also* sex chromosome.